CLEANSE & PURIFY THYSELF

"… and I will exalt thee to
the throne of power."

BOOK 1

The Cleanse

**Highly Effective Intestinal Cleansing
Removes Pounds of Dis-ease-Causing Toxins
and Dis-ease-Causing Negative Emotions**

*Some will use this program to help heal their body;
some will use it to sharpen their minds; and others
will use it to achieve their highest potential,
and that is to
love all life unconditionally.*

RICH ANDERSON, N.D., N.M.D.

**For more information see Dr. Anderson's Web Site
(http://www.cleanse . net).**

Dedicated

To the Source of All Life – our Divine Mother and Father – and all the Sons of God who have purified themselves before us and have come back to help us do likewise; also to all the strong, wonderful souls who are willing to purify themselves so that they may be Instruments of Love.

Dedicated Also

To those who read this book, are encouraged by it, and demonstrate the wisdom and strength to cleanse and purify as they strive for honesty, integrity, and love – though we may not have met, you are my brother, or sister. We are friends and more, and I pray that you will also be rewarded along your path with experiences of love such as this story records. Together we work to make this world a better place to live.

I thank God for the presence of these undaunted lights of mankind.

© Original Copyright, 1988
Current Copyright, 2000
Rich Anderson, N.D., N.M.D.
First edition, August 1987
First revision, March 1988
Major revision, July 2000
Second Edition, January 2002

Final Editing by G. Renee Getreu
Published by Christobe Publishing
P.O. Box 1643,
Medford, OR 97501

Photographers

Rich Anderson
Medford, Oregon
(pg 40-43; 205)

From: Leventhal, R., Cheadle R.
*Medical Parasitology: A
Self-Instructional Text*, 4/e. F. A.
Davis, Philadelphia, 1996, with permission.
(page 72)

Illustrators

Dr. Leonard Mehlmauer, H.P.
Camarillo, California
(page 95)

Michelle Fridkin
Tucson, Arizona
(page 98)

From: Holt, John G., ed., *Bergey's Manual of Systematic Bacteriology, Vol. 2*, Williams and Wilkins, Baltimore, Maryland, 1986, with permission. (page 134)

THE CLEANSE:
Deep, Effective Intestinal Cleansing

The *Cleanse and Purify Thyself* Book series presents
a method of self-healing and achieving
exceptional health Mother Nature's Way*
through
complete intestinal cleansing
and digestive rejuvenation.

The intestinal tract and digestive system
serve as the hub of the entire body –
all organs, glands, and even our brains, heart, and cells
are totally dependent upon a well-functioning
digestive system.

The purpose of this book is to encourage you to *CLEANSE* yourself. And then – yes, *then* – to replace it all, with unconditional love and joy, for everyone and everything. This is not medical advice, nor a prescription, just good uncommon sense. You clean out your home, you clean out your car, and it is far more important and beneficial to your well-being to clean yourself, from the inside out.

* God made Mother Nature.

TABLE OF CONTENTS

11

CHAPTER 1

MAY THE TRUTH BE KNOWN

"There is a principle which is a bar against all information, which is a proof against all argument, and which cannot fail to keep a man in everlasting ignorance. That principle is condemnation before investigation."

– Herbert Spencer

If an angel came and gave a formula that would cure almost any dis-ease, it would be against the law to claim its effectiveness. But, explaining in simple terms how we destroy our own bodies and minds and how we may reverse that destruction, leaving out all claims, will hopefully not offend the AMA, FDA, or the drug companies; will it? Though our freedom of choice in selecting the treatments we believe in to heal our bodies has largely been taken from us, we fortunately live in a country that still has the remnants of freedom of speech.

Unfortunately, people in this country are not invited to use a system of healing that has proven to be effective in reversing and preventing chronic and degenerative dis-eases. Our society has been designed to support the increase of sickness, rather than health. Every effective method that can accentuate true health is met with inexorable obstacles initiated by an invisible tyrannical influence. Truly, our society blindly follows the self-destructive precepts that lead to the declining health of our nation. Living the lifestyles that lead to rampant dis-ease is the vogue, and most people dread to be out of style. In fact they are terribly discouraged from doing so, oftentimes by force. **For beneficial lifestyles do not produce the massive profits that the creators of our modern medical system desire to generate,** and a truly effective system could interfere with the consistent increase of that flow of profits. The health profession makes money on the sick, not the healthy. **If there were a system that perpetuated radiant health, there would be little use for this book, or the vast, multi-trillion-dollar conventional (allopathic)** medical system. How sincerely do those who follow conventional medicine want people to heal?

Evidence clearly reveals: no matter what the dis-ease, as long as a person has a health-promoting attitude – a strong desire to be healthy, the willingness to do whatever is necessary to achieve good health, the relentless determined drive to seek out the truth, the discipline to apply relevant knowledge, and the willingness to forgive and love – he or she *will* bring into his or her experience that which is desired. If only health professionals would espouse this truth, the door would open for the making of a healthy nation. Too often people lose hope because their doctor tells them that there isn't a cure, and in many cases they are told that there is no hope for survival, that they are doomed to a premature death. This is a common occurrence in the medical profession simply because the medical profession uses methods that are designed to modify symptoms rather than eliminate cause – thereby ignoring diet, nutrition, toxins, congestion and the mind, emotions, and the soul. This prevents permanent healing and perpetuates a fat income.

When doctors tell their patients that there is no hope and that they are doomed to die, they have placed the seed of death in the subconscious mind of their gullible victims. They have vanquished all hope, which, by the way, is the most powerful immune builder known to science. And if their potential victims are ignorant of their own innate and awesome power to initiate total healing, then those seeds of death are likely to materialize. Indeed, when a medical doctor tells a patient that he or she has only a few weeks or months to live, **the doctor is really issuing a warning about his own treatments.** Truthfully, he is saying, "If you choose to follow my treatment plan, you will die." Now, if the patient *chooses* to follow the very program that the doctor admits will kill rather than save, death is certainly probable. I have trouble imagining why anyone would fail to seek alternatives when life depends upon it. Do these people want to die? Or have they been deeply and completely programmed?

There is no such thing as an incurable disease. But there are people who have learned to deny their own awesome creative power, and thus fail to apply it! No matter what the dis-ease, no matter how terrible it has become, or the stage of its development, someone has risen above it and found the remedy. In fact there has never been a dis-ease that someone hasn't conquered. There have been tens of thousands of people considered incurable, some even in the latter stages of dying, who suddenly and 'miraculously' became well. Even in the so-called latter stages, when there appeared no hope, people have reversed the condition and gone on to live healthy happy lives. Except for their actions, there was nothing unique about them. We all have the innate ability to overcome any dis-ease, but we must use effective methods – we must remove the cause and feed the body the nutrition it needs.

The Four Steps in Overcoming Dis-ease

The **first** step in overcoming dis-ease is to put a stop to its cause. This *always* begins by changing the habitual patterns of thoughts and feelings, which had been the invisible primal antecedent – the core cause. For, the decomposition of the body (or dying) *begins* with "suicidal" thoughts and feelings – that is, feelings of hate, anger, fear, criticism, condemnation, judgment, blame, self-pity, jealousy, resentment, and depression. These conditions decrease the life and energy within. Good health requires good thoughts and good feelings. Love, peace, harmony, poise, gratitude, and praise expand the life and light in the body, building energy, vitality and happiness. One must be at peace with one's inner self. We must face our denials and develop honesty, and integrity, and also eliminate selfishness.

The **second** step toward perfect health of the body is to stop ingesting anything, including food, that does not contain enzymes, life-force and vital nutrients. In other words, avoid putting into your mouth anything other than fresh, raw foods, since cooked and frozen foods are lifeless or dead "foods" and they cause mucus, toxins, congestion, and excess acids. Excess acids are responsible for congestion of the intestinal tract; thence unto the rest of the body. This substance is known as "mucoid plaque"[1] and significantly contributes to over 90% of *all* dis-ease – even dis-ease of the mind and heart. For, the digestive tract is the hub of the body, upon which every cell and organ depends.

The **third** step toward overcoming dis-ease is to remove the congestion, toxins, acids, and everything else, from anywhere and everywhere within the body and mind, that contributes towards dis-ease. Some health professionals choose to address only the local area of obvious trouble alone. But, as Dr. Bernard Jensen likes to say, "If you step on a cat's tail, it's the other end that yells!" Indeed, **there is no single part of the body that is not affected by the whole, and visa versa.** So, all congestion, toxins, and negativity *must be* removed, and it should begin with the removal of the mucoid plaque.

The **fourth** step toward lasting health is to then supply the body with *all* the needed elements. This includes life-force, enzymes, essential nutrients, and positive thoughts. And most important of all is love – and

---

[1] The subject of mucoid plaque is discussed in Chapter 3 of this book.

lots of it. But it is extremely difficult to successfully complete this step until the third step has been accomplished, or is well on its way.

Nature's Own Remedy – A Logical Process

Isn't this sensible? This logical process (the above four steps) is Nature's own remedy, and it is within the grasp of each one of us, yet it is almost entirely neglected by health professionals. This explains the uncountable failures, for even when there is success in curing one ailment, it is rarely more than a brief time before the "patient" develops another ailment. This is because the symptom alone was treated, not the cause, not the mind, not the subconscious, and not the soul.

The present medical treatments for chronic and degenerative dis-ease are a contemptible disgrace, especially with heart dis-ease and cancer. One prominent cancer researcher, Dr. Hardin Jones, said, *"My studies have proved conclusively that untreated cancer victims actually live up to four times longer than treated individuals... Beyond a shadow of a doubt, radical surgery on cancer patients does more harm than good."* Many medical studies, and even textbooks, verify Dr. Jones' findings. For an example, Yamada reveals in his medical textbook that there **is no indication at all that patients treated with chemotherapy have any increase of survival.**[2] He also explains **that even in cases where tumors respond to treatments, there is no indication of living longer.** Then why use it? A medical textbook on hematology reveals that the use of chemotherapy for several dis-eases **has caused serious, and often fatal, results.** This textbook explains that **the "major risk" is the** *treatment* **rather than the dis-ease.**[3] Imagine, if you will, having a serious dis-ease that results in a high percentage of fatality, and then being treated with chemicals that cause an even higher fatality rate than the dis-ease. Now, does that make any sense at all?

> *Modern medical science is the only system that advocates using treatments that are worse than the dis-ease.*

According to Edward Griffin, author of *World Without Cancer* (a revealing and stimulating book that I urge you to read), when skin cancer is

---

[2] T. Yamada, ed., *Textbook of Gastroenterology*, Yamada, T., ed., (Philadelphia, PA: J.P. Lippincott Co., 1991), pg. 1803-04.

[3] Richard Lee, M.D.; Thomas Bithell; M.D., John Forester, M.D.; John Athens, M.D.; John Lukens, M.D.; *Wintrobe's Clinical Hematology*, (Philadelphia, PA: Lea & Febiger, 1993), pg. 1744.

excluded, the average cure rate of cancer by medical doctors is 17%. Would you take your car to a mechanic if he claimed a mere 17% cure rate of transmissions? I would suggest it is time to consider other methods.[4]

The medical religion claims no cure for cancer and, what's more, no one else can either. It's against the law – even for those who know the cure. Therefore, I hereby announce that *I do not claim that my Program will cure cancer.* Should you find your cancer disappearing when you use this system, I will not accept responsibility. You'll have to take the credit yourself.[5]

The cure of cancer or any other dis-ease *has been known for decades* among a few rare health experts who understand dis-ease and its cause. But, it is also unlawful, in most states, for those experts to treat cancer unless they are M.D.s. And even the M.D.s who do understand are greatly hampered by our government and our medical authorities. What a crime against the American people! To think that there are those who can more adequately treat cancer by using non-conventional methods, but who are not legally permitted to do so!

I had better be careful here. I had better not say that all cancers can be cured. No dis-ease is curable if it's gone too far, or if the patient's attitude will not permit healing. But based on my studies and the people I've known who have conquered cancer, heart dis-ease, diabetes, and leukemia, and based on the numerous books I've read and health professionals I've talked to, the following is undeniably true: America must look to alternative healing methods if it wants to return to the healthy

---

[4] In 1999, my staff researched statistical data from the National Cancer Institute to determine their actual percentages of success with allopathic cancer treatments. After meticulously struggling through hundreds of pages of decoys, it became clear that they were hiding the true facts with ingenious ploys. Finally, after weeks of work, we were able to see through their deceptions. We found that allopathic treatments for cancer were 19% effective; however, that also included nonfatal cancers. Therefore, we were unable to determine the exact percentage, but it must be somewhere between 5% and 19%. For more information read *UnCreating Dis-ease,* by Dr. Rich Anderson, (Mt. Shasta, CA: Christobe Publishing, Projected Publication, 2002).

[5] This statement was not intended to suggest that this program would cure cancer. Only the body cures. My observations indicate to me that other treatments are necessary to successfully treat cancer. However, I believe that cleansing the bowel and removing all toxins is one of the most important steps towards strengthening the immune system and assisting the body to heal itself.

nation it once was. There are some shocking governmental statistics to support this statement.

Some Facts

The U.S. Public Health Service revealed the rate of health deterioration of the American people. Out of 100 participating nations of the world, America *was* the healthiest in 1900. In 1920, we dropped to the second highest nation. During World War II, we went back to number one - that's when sugar and meat were hard to obtain and family vegetable gardens were common. In 1978, we dropped to 79th. In 1980, we were *95th*! In 1987 we hit rock-bottom − that's number 100 on the list.[6] Yet we are said to be the wealthiest nation in the world. Are we also the most gullible? *Who,* or *what,* is responsible?[7] Here are some clues as to what may be responsible.

Leading Causes of Death in U.S. in 1996[8]

All causes	2,262,903
1. Heart dis-ease	733,834
2. Cancer	544,278
3. **Medical drugs**	**162,556**[9]
4. Stroke	160,140
5. **Infections in hospitals**	**150,000**[10]
6. Lung dis-ease	106,140
7. Accidents	93,874
8. Pneumonia/Influenza	82,579

---

[6] The U.S. Public Health Service. Quoted in "Health Realities," by Queen and Company. Also: Victor Earl Irons, Sr., *The Destruction of Your Own Natural Protective Mechanism*, (Kansas City, MO: V.E. Irons, Inc., 1995). Distributors of the Irons book may be reached at (800) 544-8147.

[7] *Ibid.*

[8] The source of all figures, except as indicated, is the National Center for Health Statistics through U.S. Department of Health & Human Services Center for Disease Control.

[9] See the Web Page of Earl Mindell, Ph.D., (www.drearlmindell.com).

[10] *Journal of Community Health*, 1980; Spring; Vol.5, No. 3., pg. 149-158. Note: Figures for after 1980 have not been released.

9. **Iatrogenic dis-ease** (Dr.-caused)	**80,000**[11]
10. Diabetes	61,559
11. HIV/AIDS	32,655
12. Suicide	30,862
13. Liver dis-ease	25,135

Total admitted **conventional medicine *caused* deaths** in 1996 was 392,556, which equals 17.34% of the deaths in America. Is this figure accurate? No, not by any means, for it does not include the many deaths caused by *failure to treat cause* and secondary side effects from medications!

Editor's Note: *Throughout this book series, three types of bullets are used. A box bullet denotes information or instructions, a diamond bullet indicates warning information, and a star shows benefits or blessings.*

More scary true facts include the following.
Please check the boxes that you would like to see changed:

❑ Over **2,556 deaths a year are caused by the use of over-the-counter drugs!**

❑ In the last 10 years, **more than 18 million Americans suffered serious, toxic side effects from medical drugs and had to be hospitalized.** That number now averages over 2 million Americans a year![12] (Talk about perpetuating profits.)

❑ 1/3 of the people admitted to hospitals are there because of the toxic effects of medications, and nearly 700,000 Americans die each year of secondary side effects from medications.[13]

---

[11] The home page of the organization: American Iatrogenic Association (http://www.aia.iatrogenic.org) It is stated on this home page that this statistic is from *Time Magazine.* American Iatrogenic Association, 2513 S. Gessner, #232, Houston, TX   77063.

[12] Reported in "Health Realities", by Queen and Company. It is stated this information is from *U.S. News and World Report.* **Even more current information, which confirms the conclusion that medical drugs are extremely dangerous, is reflected in further statistics** that have recently come to my attention.   See Rick Weiss (Washington Post Staff Writer), **"Correctly Prescribed Drugs Take Heavy Toll,"** *Washington Post* , 1998; April 15, pg. A-1.

[13] Guylaine Lanctot, M.D., *The Medical Mafia*, (Coaticook, Quebec, Canada: Here's The Key, Inc., 1995), pg. 33.

❑ About 90% of the patients who visit doctors have conditions that will either improve on their own or that are out of reach of modern medicine's ability to solve.[14]

❑ Compared to home births, babies born in hospitals are 6 times more likely to suffer distress during labor and delivery, 8 times more likely to get caught in the birth canal, 4 times more likely to need resuscitation, 4 times more likely to become infected, and 30 times more likely to be permanently injured; and mothers who give birth in hospitals are 3 times more likely to hemorrhage.[15]

❑ About 90% of surgery is unnecessary.[16]

❑ Known and admitted American deaths caused by conventional medicine is 6.77 times more than the W.W.II annual American casualities. (Are Americans at war with medical doctors and/or drug companies? Imagine a war where one side doesn't have enough sense to know that their enemies are killing them. And if that isn't bad enough, imagine that the side that is losing is financially and socially supporting their enemies in their own destruction and encouraging their friends, families, and even their children to do the same! Has our society gone totally insane or is it just deeply programmed?)

❑ It is estimated that *over* **1000 babies, in America alone, die from DPT** vaccine *EVERY YEAR* **and over 12,000 are** *permanently* **damaged;** and approximately **20% of American children suffer from a "developmental disability"**[17] **as a result of vaccines –** *EVERY YEAR!*.[18] Pressure from parents who had experienced death and disability of their children from vaccines caused Congress to adopt the *National Childhood Vaccination*

[14] T. A Brennan, et al., "Incidence of Adverse Event and Negligence in Hospitalized Patients. Results of the Harvard Medical Practice Study," *New England Journal of Medicine*, 1991; Feb 7, pg. 370-376.

[15] Robert S. Mendelsohn, M.D., *Confessions of a Medical Heretic*, (Chicago, IL: Contemporary Books, 1979), pg. 91.

[16] Ibid., pg. 49.

[17] The term "developmental disability" is commonly used to include mentally retardation, blindness, deafness, autistism, epilepsy, learning-disabilities, and emotional instability. Future juvenile delinquents, career criminals, those demonstrating abnormal social behaviors, and those who are immune deficient may also be categorized as developmentally disabled.

[18] Harris L. Coulter, *Vaccination Social Violence and Criminality: The Medical Assault on the American Brain*, (Berkeley, Calif.: North Atlantic Books, 1990), pg. xii – xiv.

Compensation Law authorizing payment of damages to children harmed by immunization. However, they conveniently forgot to convey this knowledge to the public and apparently to doctors who administer vaccines. See Appendix II for more information about vaccination compensation. [19]

Almost on a daily basis, we are all exceedingly impressed with the incredible achievements in the field of medical surgery. But in other fields, such as in the treatments for chronic and degenerative dis-ease, the crimes against life are endless as the above atrocities indicate. Investigation reveals succinctly and emphatically that the medical industry has succumbed to the hypnotic temptations of wealth, power, and vanity. It is obviously in the best interest of conventional medicine for practitioners to remain blind to efficient remedies. Yes, even at the cost of ceaseless suffering and death of millions of people and innocent creatures of God. The fault is not with the millions of doctors, nurses, and others who do their best to alleviate suffering. The enemy is the system and the money-mongers who manipulate and perpetuate it. Most doctors and their staffs are outstanding and compassionate individuals, and we need to recognize this. They do what they do because they were taught to do so, just as the majority of society has also accepted the illusions that conventional medicine is a benefit for everyone. It's time for our programmed and brainwashed society to awaken. In the process of awakening, we must remember to remain calm and not allow ourselves to become overly angered by what we may see.

---

[19] Many people consider the vaccination of children the worst crime in the history of mankind. Vaccines may be one of the primary causes of the explosion of dis-ease in the Western World. Vaccines are unnatural toxic filth, and it has recently been discovered that they mutate the immune system into impotency. No one really knows how many people have died from vaccines – undoubtedly millions. There is a great deal of controversy about vaccines, but those who do the research are convinced beyond a shadow of a doubt that **vaccines are far, far more harmful than the dis-eases they purportedly eliminate**. In the opinion of many doctors, scientists, and researchers, the medical propaganda about vaccines is mostly unscientific and in many cases fraudulent. There is no doubt that many thousands of children, as well as adults, are being permanently harmed, and oftentimes killed, by vaccines. This is far more common than people think. Those who wish to investigate before they receive another injection, can read some of the books about this subject listed in the Recommended Reading Section at the back of this book. Take away the profit made from vaccines, and vaccines would disappear. Vaccines are not beneficial except perhaps in a few rare instances; they do, however, benefit those who make and sell them.

A Departure from Nature

Since 1900, the basic, sensible theories of health care have changed dramatically. The major change was the shift from natural to unnatural: from using harmless and beneficial herbs to unnatural and harmful drugs. Accompanying this shift was the onset of processed foods; the use of preservatives and other unnatural chemicals sprayed on food, especially herbicides and pesticides[20] (deadly poisons); polluted air; and chlorinated and fluoridated water[21]; and now electronic poisoning. This unnatural approach to life has had its detrimental effect not only upon the American people, but the entire world.

In my opinion, as long as our approach to healing, except in rare cases, involves the use of drugs, chemicals, radiation, and scalpels, true health will never be obtained. If we sincerely want to bring the American people back to health, or if we personally wish to reclaim our own perfect health, we must stop using drugs and chemicals that pollute, suppress, and weaken our bodies. We must return to the natural methods that our Creator designed and created; and that obviously means using herbs and other natural methods that cleanse, purify, and strengthen the body.[22]

---

[20] The active ingredient of pesticides is arsenic – a deadly poison.

[21] Chlorine in water is now known to cause cancer. Chlorine was created in World War I for use in gas warfare. Fluoride is a deadly poison, even more deadly than lead. Sodium fluoride is harmful to teeth and the mind. Calcium fluoride is the only fluoride that is beneficial for teeth. Unfortunately, and evidently without complete investigation, the FDA approved fluoridation, and *sodium* fluoride, rather than *calcium* fluoride, was added to the water systems of major American cities. Eventually the truth came out: the use of sodium fluoride in tap water led to an increase of tooth decay, a 12% increase of Mongoloid children, and a massive increase of Alzheimer's disease. There is evidence that sodium fluoride not only dulls the mind but also makes one susceptible to suggestion. Now that the facts are known, why isn't the FDA doing something to stop its use?

[22] This is not to say that we should never use drugs or surgery, but that we should use them only with great discretion and as a last resort, and only when we are certain that nothing else can work (this would be rare, if natural healing were used properly). But there are times when only a drug will stop pain, and there are times that coffee enemas stop pain better than any drug. But this entire situation has become terribly out of hand, and millions of people die unnecessarily, and many more millions suffer because of it.

CHAPTER 2

A GREAT KEY TO HEALTH: ORGANIC ELECTROLYTES

"Man does not die, he kills himself."

– Seneca

"Vitality and beauty are gifts of nature for those who live according to its laws."

– Leonardo DaVinci

Following breathing, and the heart beating, the next most important physiological function our bodies perform is the maintaining of a balanced pH.[23] Regulation of pH is essential because every enzyme system, cell, organ, and gland in the body is influenced by pH. Excluding accidents and genetic weakness, dis-ease often begins to occur after we have altered our normal pH balance and become deficient in minerals, especially organic electrolyte minerals[24] – not minerals from rock, but minerals from organic matter (plants).[25]

Even when a slight depletion of any of the electrolytes occurs, many of our organs and glands become severely challenged, weakened, toxic, and sluggish, for only slight changes in pH from normal levels can cause extreme alterations in the rates of chemical reactions – inside and outside of our cells. Any depletion means that health is plummeting and

---

[23] pH is the symbol for "potential hydrogen" and is used with a number to indicate levels of acidity or alkalinity. The greater the amount of hydrogen atoms, the stronger the acid, and the lower the pH number. Anything from 0 - 7, indicates acidity. The more diminished the amount of hydrogen atoms, the more increased the alkalinity and, the higher the number.

[24] Sodium, potassium, calcium, magnesium, lithium, and phosphorus are the main electrolytes that the body uses.

[25] The body cannot efficiently use rock minerals. It must use the minerals that have passed through the plant kingdom. Minerals from the plant kingdom have been chelated to a protein molecule through the magic of photosynthesis.

healing is significantly inhibited until the depletion has been rectified. Depletion also means that acids are accumulating. And acids are harmful to the body. When people become too over-acid they may die in a coma, and when they become too over-alkaline they could die of tetany or convulsions. At a certain point between the two, we have health, but if the pH of our blood, of any organ, or of any cell moves toward one of these extremes, dysfunction and dis-ease are *always* the result.

Key Points to Digestion

When we eat, we chew the food and it goes into the stomach. Here it is saturated by hydrochloric acid (HCl). HCl has an extreme acid pH of .5 (point 5). This is the only place in the body that needs to be acid. This low pH activates pepsinogen enzymes, which are essential for efficient digestion of protein. After the stomach has completed its digestive phase, it releases the chyme through the pyloric valve. (Chyme is a mixture of food, stomach acids, and enzymes.) The food (chyme) is now highly acidic and as it enters the duodenum, it is saturated by large amounts of alkaline fluids from the Brunner glands, bile, and pancreatic juices. To maintain good health, it is absolutely essential that our intestines maintain an alkaline environment; for the pancreatic and the other 22 intestinal enzymes **can only function optimally in a pH above 7**. Not only that, before the body can absorb the food into the bloodstream and use it, it must bring the food up to a 7.4 pH, for the blood always maintains a 7.4 pH.

Physiological Control of pH

Our bodies have several incredible control mechanisms to assure pH control. One process is called the buffer system. By eliminating complex explanations, we can say that the first step is for the body to buffer the acids by absorbing the acid with the electrolyte *organic sodium* and bicarbonate. Each time an acid is buffered by the sodium, the pH rises. In this process the body brings the acids to a level in which it can safely remove them from the body through the kidneys and control pH. **But each time an electrolyte is used to buffer acids, the electrolyte is removed – lost forever**.

The more acids we consume, especially from acid-forming foods, the greater the potential of an electrolyte deficiency. A key to good health is to eat enough food that has a greater amount of electrolytes than acids – alkaline-forming food. For when we eat too much acid-forming food, we drain our bank account of electrolytes. We can also become electrolyte-deficient from emotional stress. Whether we lose electrolytes via stress or from acid-forming foods matters not; once our electrolyte storehouse is depleted, declining health is inevitable and one problem after another develops. And too much depletion means death, for our bodies cannot live without adequate electrolytes.

A Missing Key in Overcoming Illness

With this understanding, it becomes obvious that **the most important factor in treating *any* dis-ease** is to supply the body with the organic electrolyte minerals that it lacks and that it unequivocally needs for regeneration. **Without a full supply of electrolytes, our bodies cannot maintain themselves, much less heal themselves.** And yet **99% of doctors never give it a thought**; and even if they did, only a few have the understanding necessary to correct this serious dis-ease-threatening profile. This medical neglect has caused the premature death of millions of people and perpetuated the dis-ease and suffering of many millions more. It also perpetuates the medical industry and helps reduce the overpopulation of the world. So maybe there is a reason for this abject neglect.

Most people in America have already lost this delicate health-essential balance and are moving first towards over-acidity and then on to alkalinity. **Both over-acidity and over-alkalinity are due to a lack of electrolytes, particularly *organic* sodium, and never because of an overabundance of electrolytes**[26]. Another important point is that long before anyone nears death's door because of an electrolyte deficiency, that person usually has contracted various dis-ease conditions, which most people are totally unaware of until the malady has progressed into pain, tiredness, or some other symptom.

The Difference Between Alkaline-forming and Acid-forming Foods

Alkaline-forming foods contain an abundance of the electrolytes needed to buffer acids in the food, and help build the body's reserve. Acid-

---

[26] Doctors know that to correct acidity we need alkalinity, but some misinformed doctors believe that to correct alkalosis, acids must be given. Many deaths have resulted from this mistake. Though there are several caues of alkalosis, I am referring to alkalosis that occurs with chronic dis-ease, and this is caused by excess acids and a lack of sodium. See A. C. Guyton, *Textbook of Medical Physiology*, 7th edition, (Philadelphia, PA: W. B. Saunders Co, 1986), pg. 447.

forming foods do not. Acid-forming food forces the body to retrieve the buffering electrolytes from its own reserve. The same thing occurs with stress. Stress creates acids, and stress has no electrolytes at all. Both acid-forming food and stress cause a deficit in the body's reserve, which is needed for exercise, thinking, coping with illness, and healing.

Organic Sodium

You may wonder how Americans become deficient in sodium, for most people add sodium chloride (table salt) to almost every meal they eat. This is vital to understand. **Sodium chloride (table salt), cannot be used by the body.** Minerals from rock have no protein and are therefore highly caustic and toxic to our bodies. Too much potassium chloride, for example, can kill you. Sodium chloride is so toxic that it can increase blood pressure and is an irritant to cell membranes, and cannot be used efficiently in the buffer system or in our cells. The body can only efficiently use sodium that has been chelated to a protein molecule. Minerals chelated like this are referred to as "organic."

It is quite obvious to some doctors, although the conventional medical profession has not acknowledged it, that sodium chloride cannot be used in metabolism. This has been proven by clinical studies. One study revealed that when sodium chloride was given to individuals who are prone to hypertension, their blood pressure rose, **but when *organic sodium* was given to these same people, their blood pressure moved towards normal**. It was also found that **sodium chloride induced the body to lose calcium, whereas *organic* sodium induced a decrease in calcium loss**. An interesting fact arose in this study that completely baffled the researchers. **Whenever sodium chloride was ingested, the body quickly removed it. However, when *organic* sodium was given, the body held it.** Why? You should by now have the answer, but if you do not, please reread this chapter. The answer, however, is that the body could not use the sodium chloride because it is toxic and unusable; therefore it discarded it as quickly as possible even though it was deficient in *organic* sodium. But it will retain the *organic* sodium because it desperately needs it.[27, 28]

---

[27] Theodore W. Kurtz, M.D.; Hamoundi A. Al-Bander, M.D.; R. Curtis Morris Jr., M.D., "Salt-Sensitive Essential Hypertension In Men," *New England Journal Of Medicine,* Vol. 317, No. 17, pg. 1043-1048.

[28] Lindsay H. Allen, Ph.D.; E. A., Oddoye, Ph.D.; and S. Margen, M.D., "Salt-Sensitive Essential Hypercalciuria; A Longer Term Study," *The American Journal of Clinical Nutrition,* 1979; April; Issue 32, pg. 741-749.

How Electrolyte Deficiency Causes Dis-ease

As I said, when the body becomes low in its supply of an electrolyte such as *organic* sodium, **it is forced to go to another part of its self to retrieve the electrolyte**, and it will do this even if it has to **kill its own cells.** This statement should shock you, awaken you, and ring many bells within. For here is a major key to most chronic and degenerative diseases. Remember, the body absolutely must have electrolytes to survive, and any deficiency means chemical imbalance, cellular dysfunction, a decline in health, and the inability to heal.

The Destruction of the Digestive System

When the body is forced to retrieve *organic* sodium from within itself, the most benign and efficient pathway is the bile. This way it can avoid having to directly injure itself. However, **the removal of sodium from bile, though harmless in the beginning, has a devastating chain reaction.**

The removal of sodium from bile causes the bile pH to drop. The more it drops, the more acid it becomes. When bile drops to a certain point, gallstones are formed.[29,30] As you know, gallstones can cause severe problems, including life-threatening afflictions.

When bile becomes acid, it is highly caustic and irritates the intestinal wall. Bile can become so acid that it can burn a hole right through the gut wall; in fact, 90% of all so-called "stomach" or "peptic" ulcers are found in the duodenum near the bile duct.[31] Bile irritation is associated with development of polyps, bowel tumors, Colon cancer, irritable bowel syndrome (IBS), leaky gut syndrome, and various other bowel "dis-eases."

Fortunately the body has a protective mechanism that can help to compensate for this dangerous scenario – mucin secretion. Mucin is a glycoprotein mucus. It is secreted by intestinal glands and can line the

---

[29] In comparing the composition of bile to the composition of cholesterol gallstones, we find that the only difference between the two is that gallstones lack sodium and potassium.

[30] The highest rates of gallstone dis-ease are in countries where diets are high in animal protein. Conversely, the lowest rates are in countries where diets are mostly vegetarian.

[31] Wynn Kapit, Robert Macey, and Esmail Meisami, *The Physiology Coloring Book*, (Philadelphia, PA: Harper Collins Publishers, 1987), pg. 78.

intestines, thereby protecting it from acids and other irritants. Mucin is the primal essence of mucoid plaque.

The consequences of acid bile and mucoid plaque include the following: poor digestion, poor assimilation, toxic accumulation, poor peristalsis, mutation or destruction of friendly bacteria, bowel dis-eases, and the commencement of many chronic and degenerative dis-eases. And all this is caused primarily because of *organic* electrolyte deficiencies.

The next most likely locale for the body to retrieve *organic* sodium is the stomach. In a healthy person, the parietal cells of the stomach manufacture hydrochloric acid (HCl), an essential element in digestion. But in order to do this, it must have large amounts of *organic* sodium to protect the stomach cells from the HCl. And so it is at this site that we find the greatest store of *organic* sodium. However, the stomach needs this large storehouse of organic sodium, and *if it is diminished, the stomach is forced to stop HCl production.* For if the HCl production were continued without the protection of *organic* sodium, the HCl would burn a hole right through the stomach. Yes, *a lack of organic* sodium is associated with ulcers. Therefore, a lack of sodium in the stomach not only means a shutdown of HCL production, it also means that pepsinogen cannot be activated, **nor can proteins be efficiently digested.**

Lack of HCl and enzymes devastates digestion. Poor digestion always means that health is diminishing. Not only that, but a lack of the normal HCl in the stomach **allows potential pathogenic bacteria, parasites, and yeasts to enter the inter sanctum of the gastrointestinal tract.** This allows the entire body to become exposed to these pathogens. So you see, HCl has at least two highly important functions. It protects us from harmful microorganisms and helps digest our food. When HCl is unavailable, due to sodium deficiency, we become more vulnerable to dis-ease, digestion becomes inefficient, and then **even good food can become toxic.** This is a typical scenario affecting the lives of approximately 80% or more of the population in the Western World. In a private conversation, Dr. Bernard Jensen once commented to me that his research had revealed that over 80% of people who are admitted to a hospital and 100% of AIDS patients have *no* HCl production.

A few years ago, two children died from *E. coli* poisoning from eating a hamburger at one of the fast-food chains. It was very likely that they had been severely depleted of sodium and had little or no HCl production.[32] Otherwise, the HCl would have eliminated the *E. coli* while

---

[32] They probably also lacked proper bacteria in the gut, which, had it been present, could have handled the *E. coli*. I have no doubt that these children had a history of eating acid-forming foods and drink, and probably had

still in the stomach. You can be sure that most of the people who eat at such places are electrolyte-deficient and lack HCl. People who suffer from so-called food poisoning have the same problem. They lack sodium, and HCl production is inefficient. This is a common scenario with those who eat the Standard American Diet (SAD).

Other Problems Associated with Organic Sodium Deficiency

Another area where the body can retrieve sodium is the joints. **When *organic sodium* is removed from the joints, which is common, then arthritis develops.** The body can also remove sodium from the muscles. When this occurs, the muscles become weak and flabby. When *organic sodium* is removed from the liver, the liver becomes weak and inefficient.[33] Many serious difficulties can develop from liver weakness, such as skin problems, headaches, pains, poor eyesight, depression, mental problems, sugar problems, allergies, blood sugar problems, tiredness, cancer, digestion weakness, poor memory, muscle weakness, lack of endurance, etc. The liver affects every cell and organ in the body. Almost every known dis-ease can be related to the liver.

When the body becomes severely deficient in *organic sodium*, its partner, potassium, can also become deficient. A severe deficiency of *organic* sodium automatically depletes potassium; in fact, **it may be impossible to be potassium-deficient unless an *organic sodium* deficiency is present.**[34] Potassium is abundant in most foods, especially fruits and vegetables. It is almost impossible to be deficient in potassium unless one of the following is true: 1) you don't eat, 2) you can't digest food, or 3) you are deficient in sodium.[35]

---

antibiotics treatment, which destroyed their normal intestinal bacteria. What really killed them – the *E. coli* or the antibiotics and acid-forming food?

[33] You can test for *organic sodium* in the liver by using pH papers. If your saliva pH is 6.3 or less, your liver is deficient. If it is less than 6.1, your profile indicates danger. See Chapter 11 in this book.

[34] The body demands a specific ratio of sodium to potassium. When sodium is low, the body secretes the hormone aldosterone, which triggers the body to reabsorb sodium, but when there is insufficient sodium, aldosterone forces the body to release potassium into the urine, thereby achieving its proper ratio. Guyton, pg. 911.

[35] Symptoms of potassium deficiency include heart dis-ease, muscle aches and pains, mood swings, depression, weakness, fears, cynicism, sagging

Although calcium deficiency can develop independently of an *organic sodium* deficiency,[36] it can also be related. And when calcium becomes low, osteoporosis and other bone problems may develop.[37] Evidence indicates that when organic sodium and organic potassium deficiencies occur, that organic calcium and magnesium may be used to replace organic sodium and potassium. This could contribute towards calcium and magnesium deficiencies.[38]

The Intestines Must Be Alkaline

A fact missed by most health professionals is that intestinal enzymes can only function optimally in a pH above 7.0. This mistake is reflected by the overuse of *Lactobacillus bacteria* (*acidophilus*, etc.) and other extreme acid-producing probiotics. Though there is a need and a place for these acid-producing bacteria, in many cases they are being used excessively and people suffer as a result. I have two clinical studies in my possession that clearly show that individuals reached critical acidosis and were hospitalized from taking acidophilus. This subject is discussed further in Chapter 9: "The Powerful Ingredients of a Superb Intestinal Cleanse," under the subheading "Probiotics."

My point here is that the intestines need to be alkaline, and as long as the bowel maintains alkalinity – and we have an abundance of

---

organs, edema, suicidal impulses, sunken eyes, a sensation like sand in the eyes, dry skin, gastritis, muscular atrophy, bowel problems, eye problems, sore knees, shallow breathing, skin eruptions, liver problems, fatigue, cancer, cracked lips, nerve problems, and muscle weakness.

[36] For a thorough explanation backed by clincal studies read *Cleanse & Purify Thyself*, Book 2.

[37] Symptoms of calcium deficiency include a weak liver, tooth decay, malnutrition, blood deficiencies, hemorrhaging, hemorrhoids, muscle weakness, mental sluggishness, craving for salt and tobacco, dull headache, glandular problems, bronchial congestion, poor complexion, wrinkled skin, earaches, bloating, nervousness, inferiority complexes, uncontrolled emotions, pessimism, poor memory, desire for seclusion, shyness, mental difficulties, melancholy, moodiness, depression, frequent colds, muscles aches and cramps, poor digestion, shifting pains, cracked skin on hands or feet, and toothaches; also associated with anemia, arthritis, heart conditions, eczema, asthma, etc.

[38] Professor C. Lewis Kervran, *Biological Transmutations,* (Magalia, CA: Happiness Press, 1988), pg. 20.

electrolytes, hydrochloric acid, and a strong liver – then a good digestive system will continue throughout life. The moment our digestive system cannot function optimally, health is failing.

Do you now see now how we can *create* dis-ease? And how we become susceptible to "germs?" And how we can damage our digestive system? Remember, the digestive system is the hub of the body. Every single cell and organ depends upon this precious system. The moment our digestive system becomes inadequate, the liver and other organs and systems are challenged. If we fail to recover the full function of this essential system, then it is downhill henceforth.

Constipation and Diarrhea

As these conditions advance, constipation and/or diarrhea often develop. Diarrhea is often associated with constipation.[39] When there is constipation, there is an extremely toxic bowel, and pathogenic bacteria thrive in toxic bowel environments. When the toxicity builds to a certain degree, acids, from bacteria and/or parasites, attack the bowel mucosa, and the bowel glands flush the bowel with mucus and liquids, thereby creating diarrhea. Diarrhea can drain electrolytes quickly and create severe electrolyte deficiency. If this is not corrected quickly, death is likely. Electrolyte deficiency due to diarrhea is a leading cause of death in Third World countries.

Constipation causes the bowel to become extremely toxic, and these toxic particles enter the blood, forcing the liver and kidneys to handle excessive toxic overloads. Too much toxicity and acids from the bowel eventually weaken the liver and the gut lining. Leaky bowel syndrome develops, and then the liver, kidneys, spleen, and other organs are even more challenged. Toxins in the blood contaminate the hereditarily weak and injured areas of the body first. On and on it goes until every organ and gland is affected. How rapidly will these conditions develop? This depends upon the constitutional weakness of the body, attitudes of the mind, and the degree of indulgence in acid-forming foods and highly processed foods. It is also related to the quality of fruits and vegetables that are eaten

---

[39] Ideally, a person should have a bowel movement the first thing each morning and within 30 minutes after each meal. If three meals a day are eaten, there should be four (4) movements a day, even with light meals. Any fewer than that indicates an inclination towards constipation. Fewer than two (2) BM's daily indicates there is a health problem developing. With less than one (1) BM daily, health is plummeting rapidly.

(organically grown versus the mineral-deficient commercially grown produce). But most influential of all are the ways we think and feel.

It is rather perplexing that so few medical doctors have realized the following points[40]:

☐ Electrolytes must be organic.
☐ Most people are sodium deficient.
☐ Proper diet is essential to good health and overcoming illness.
☐ The bowel is always one of the most important systems to treat for almost every "dis-ease."
☐ Next to the bowel, the liver is the paramount organ to treat for almost every "dis-ease."
☐ *Acidophilus* should be used as a treatment, not for implants.
☐ Bile becomes acid because of a lack of organic sodium.

When proponents of conventional medicine finally do comprehend the body's need for *organic* minerals, they will be forced to acknowledge that diet does indeed play an important role in health, and then medical schools may actually begin to study nutrition.[41] This is an extremely important subject and its full understanding and application would allow healing for many who are not able to heal today. Thus it could prevent a high percentage of various "dis-eases."

MINERALS – Important Key to Health

From the above explanations, it is easy to see how we create our own dis-ease. We can also understand how important it is to consume a diet of mostly alkaline-forming foods that are grown in soil that has an abundant supply of minerals and other nutrients – in other words, organically grown. The world needs to hear this: **every single function of our bodies is dependent upon an adequate supply of minerals, and there are no exceptions**. It is critical to have enough of the right kind of minerals for life and health. With every case of chronic or degenerative disease, the mineral supply has become seriously deficient and the pH of body fluids abnormal. **Adequate healing cannot take place until we have replenished our mineral supply and brought our bodies into the balance.** Eating only organically grown produce is the only way we can be

---

[40] As noted on page 20, the "box bullets" indicate informational points.

[41] There are 125 medical schools in the U.S. Only 30 of them offer any training in nutrition, and among those 30, less than 3 hours of training are given in nutrition.

confident that we are receiving an adequate supply of minerals, since commercially grown produce is usually deficient in minerals and toxic with chemicals.[42] Studies have shown that **organically grown produce has a range of 50 to 400% more nutrition than commercially grown produce**, and significantly less lead and mercury.[43]

Editor's Note: *Throughout this book series, three types of bullets are used. A box bullet denotes information or instructions, a diamond bullet indicates warning information, and a star shows benefits or blessings.*

How We Deplete Ourselves of Minerals

♦ Negative emotions (stress)
♦ Eating too many acid-forming foods
♦ Medical drugs
♦ Poor digestion and assimilation
♦ Eating foods from inadequate soil –
  commercially grown foods
♦ Bacteria and parasite infections
♦ Dysfunctional adrenals or kidneys
♦ Shallow breathing

Ways to Maintain Health and Build Mineral Reserves

❑ Develop a happy and positive point of view
❑ Eat wholesome, organically grown fruits and vegetables
❑ Eat a diet that is 80% or more alkaline-forming food
❑ Cleanse & Purify the entire body and mind
❑ Rebuild the digestive system, then the liver and other organs
❑ Avoid drugs, vaccines, chlorine, fluoride, and other poisons
❑ Get plenty of rest and exercise
❑ Breathe deeply
❑ Form the habit of feeling sincere appreciation for the many gifts that life gives us.

---

[42] Even eating organically grown food is no guarantee that we will receive all the nutritents we need. Eating food grown in our own gardens and orchards is much more beneficial than eating any store-purchased food.

[43] B. L. Smith, "Organic Foods vs. Supermarket Foods; Element Levels," *Journal of Applied Nutrition*, 1993; 45(1), pg. 35-39.

Summary

It is vital for our bodies to maintain a perfect pH balance, and as long as they are capable of doing so, we have a very good chance of maintaining our health all through our lives. But if this balance is lost, it will be impossible to maintain good health. The further we deplete our electrolytes and move towards greater acidity, the more our bodies lose control over pH and the greater the threat to first, the digestive system; subsequently, the liver; then the immune system; and finally all the other organs. After these three systems weaken, we become susceptible to one compounding problem after another. It has been recognized that it takes 20 years to create cancer. Now you have an insight as to how this takes place.

CHAPTER 3

THE DIGESTIVE SYSTEM, AND THE CREATION OF THE DREADED MUCOID PLAQUE

"This layer of mucus, when adhering closely to the mucosal surface, probably functions as a barrier to membrane digestion and most likely also to absorption... where, with increasing age, the mucus layer becomes more pronounced and widespread. ...Furthermore, mucus on the mucosal surface inhibits contact of carbohydrates with disaccharidases, resulting in clinical intolerance of lactose or sucrose in the presence of normal disaccharidase activities."

– J. Rainer Poley M.D.

"If we desire good health, then whatever we have put into our bodies that interferes with their ability to function properly, must be removed."

– Dr. Rich Anderson

"Remember that when you help one organ, every other organ benefits also."

– Dr. Bernard Jensen

What is Mucoid Plaque?

The phrase "mucoid plaque" is a coined term that I developed to describe the complex glycoproteins secreted by intestinal glands, which form a gel-like slimy mucus layer and can coat the various hollow organs, especially the intestinal canal. In the intestines and stomach, mucoid plaque usually forms a continuous overlay. It is composed of a structured fibrillary network and is arranged in layers. "Mucoid" is a general term for mucin, mucoprotein, or glycoprotein, which is the primary constituent of mucoid plaque. "Plaque" designates a film of mucus on a surface.

Medical doctors and, surprisingly, many gastroenterologists are not trained in medical school in regard to this important subject, and many doctors have been utterly confused whenever their patients discuss mucoid plaque with them. They are, however, aware of the many altered forms that mucoid plaque transforms into – and that progress into dis-ease. But they have failed to recognize that many advanced stages of bowel dis-eases, such as diverticulitis, polyps, atrophic gastritis, cystic fibrosis, malignancy, inflammatory bowel dis-eases, peptic ulcers, intestinal metaplasia, dysplasia, bowel cancer, and others, are altered or degraded stages of mucoid plaque (mucin). Curiously, they seem to ignore that the above dis-eases **are advanced forms of something that was previously not as advanced.** Indeed, advanced stages of dis-ease were at one time not as advanced and at one time had a cause – a beginning and multiple intermediate states. Truly, dis-ease, like any other condition or process either progresses or regresses.

I say this with a bit of sarcasm because I've seen so many doctors completely disregard the early and in-between stages of dis-eases, and yet acknowledge that it takes almost 20 years for bowel cancer, etc. to develop. They seem to say that "the bowel is pure and clean *until*," – "oops, where did that come from?" Medical science acknowledges that bowel dis-eases are related to mucin, but fails to recognize that mucin accumulates in stages prior to dis-ease. Thus, conventional doctors miss that removing this mucilaginous plaque can prevent serious and even life-threatening dis-ease.

If allopathic doctors (M.D.s) were more concerned about the prevention and causes of dis-ease, and especially of the importance of cleansing the body, rather than just treating symptoms, they would long ago have delved into this extremely important subject. Those who have been seriously involved with cleansing the body cannot help but observe the almost unbelievable amounts of mucoid plaque being released from the body during serious and effective purification. Medical scientists should have looked into this about 50 years ago, because **its existence is so blatantly obvious and its removal produces such incredible benefits to the human body, mind, and spirit.** I believe that this subject was known but purposely denied because medical authorities, especially those who control medical schools' curriculum, clearly understood the importance and the effectiveness of bowel cleansing, **and also its potential to inhibit the escalation of enormous medical profits.**[44]

Clinical and anatomical studies from many scientific papers and textbooks have clearly demonstrated the existence of mucoid plaque in the alimentary canal, but the descriptions presented in these studies are nothing compared to the vivid experience of observing its exit from one's own body! My book *Cleanse & Purify Thyself*, Book 2 (previously titled: Book 1.5), describes mucoid plaque in scientific detail. It lists well over 100 medical statements and sources that describe this substance. It shows pictures of mucoid plaque both inside the body and after removal from the body. Book 2 also explains the **many different stages of mucoid plaque as it transforms or alters from one dis-ease to another – including bowel cancer.** As I said, medical science has many "dis-ease" terms to describe each condition in its advanced stages, but has nothing to describe the early and intermediate stages. Nor does it have a term that consolidates them all into one category. Hence, I created "mucoid plaque."

Mucoid plaque can line the entire alimentary canal, from the tip of the tongue and all the way to the other end. As described in Chapter 2, mucoid plaque development is generally associated with acid bile. Bile should not be acidic; in fact, bile pH should be above 8.0, which is quite alkaline. However, with most people in the Western World, especially meat-eating people, their bile pH is well below 8.0, even as low as 4.5. And this low pH is caustic – it irritates and burns the intestinal wall. In this acid environment, the gut wall is forced to protect itself and does so by secreting mucin, thereby lining the gut with a protective mucus shield. Other irritants to our alimentary canal, which can also trigger mucoid plaque, are table salt, alcohol, drugs, acid-forming bacteria, heavy metals, pathogenic microorganisms, and parasites. I explained how bile becomes acid in the last chapter; but its primary causes, acid-forming food and stress, need further emphasis. Included in acid-forming foods are grains, especially bread; cereals; sugar; soft drinks; and coffee. A major hidden cause of acid production is eating foods that the body is unable to digest. For example, I estimate that more than 50% of Americans cannot digest wheat properly,

---

[44] The following quote may be found in the article titled: "Health Costs Soaring," from *USA Today*, Monday, Dec. 30, 1991: "Total U.S. health-care spending will rise 11% next year to $817 billion, the Commerce Department predicted Sunday. The growth rate, the same as this year's, will put health spending at 14% of gross national product. The report projects health-care spending will continue to grow 12% to 13% a year for the next five years, putting it at roughly $1.5 trillion by 1997."

and it is known that more than 50% cannot digest milk.[45] For a more complete list of acid-forming foods, see the chart on acid- and alkaline-forming foods in the back of the book.

When people continue to live the lifestyles that cause bile to become acid, mucoid plaque production continues without reprieve, and of course it continues to build, becoming thicker, firmer, and more widespread. Clinical studies have clearly shown this to be true.[46] The accumulated mucoid plaque may be several inches thick, but in most areas of the gut, it is probably less than one-quarter of an inch thick. It occurs in the stomach, as well as on the entire surface of both the small and large intestines. Even the health care professionals, enlightened as to the benefits of cleansing, generally consider only the four to six feet of the colon, ignoring the 22 feet of the small intestine, and the stomach. Especially the small intestine is critical for full digestion, and absorption of nutrients.

Because most people are in the habit of eating toxic high-protein (acid-forming) foods with each meal, and often in between, bowel problems and mucoid plaque development in the meat-eating world are epidemic, along with gallstones, arthritis, rheumatism, heart dis-ease, cancer, chronic fatigue, mental and emotional problems, and many related disorders. It is important to know that **mucoid plaque appears to be the forerunner of many, many dis-ease conditions. Not just in the bowel, but dis-eases throughout the entire body.** This fact cannot be overemphasized. Continuous ingestion of acid-forming foods and unnatural, processed, so-called foods causes a gradual increase of mucoid plaque, which becomes thicker, firmer, and increasingly toxic – the perfect breeding ground of armies of pathogenic microorganisms and parasites. It becomes like the city dump, full of unbelievable amounts of filth.

Mucoid plaque is also highly adhesive, and therefore the reversal of this condition seldom, if ever, occurs during one's lifetime. Unfortunately, even the people who have changed their diets and eat only raw fruits and vegetables **still have mucoid plaque clinging to their bowels until they take the necessary steps to remove it.** And fortunately, **with the use of specific herbs in specific combinations, the body can release the mucoid plaque, layer after layer.**

---

[45] Lactose intolerance is found in more than 70% of black Americans, Orientals, Arabs, Greeks, Eskimos, Indians, Africans, and Asians, and in more than 50% of white Americans. Yamada, pg. 1521.

[46] J. Rainier Poley, "The Scanning Electron Microscope: How Valuable in the Evaluation of Small Bowel Mucosal Pathology in Chronic Childhood Diarrhea?" *Journal of Pediatric Gastroenterology and Nutrition*, 1991; May-June; 7(3), pg. 386-394.

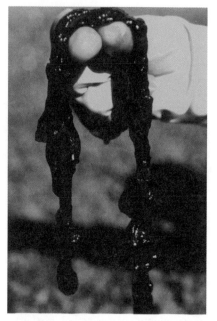

Black Mucoid Plaque from Colon

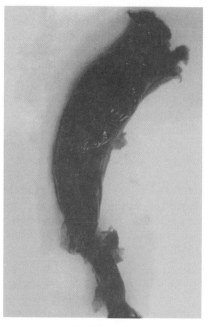

Brown Mucoid Plaque from Jejunum
Note the long, fairly straight and
shallow creases running lengthwise
along the surface of the plaque.

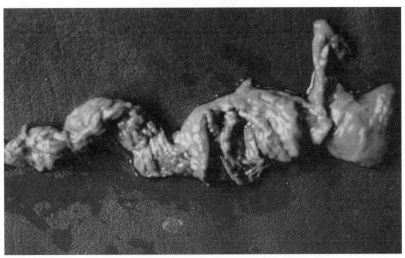

Yellow Mucoid Plaque from Upper Ileum

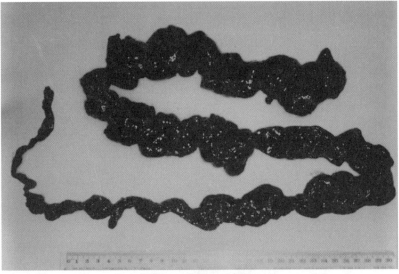

Long Piece of Mucoid Plaque.
Note the distorted shape and narrowing of the alimentary canal.

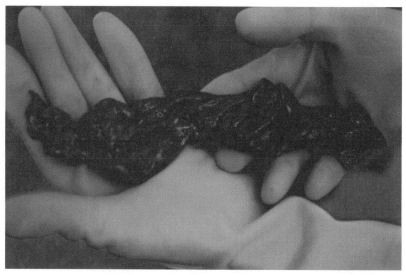

Colon Plaque—Stiff Segment
(Drier, harder and more leather-like)

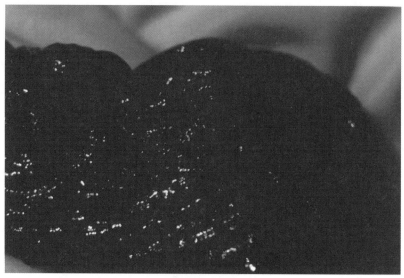

Pile of Plaque
(Softer)

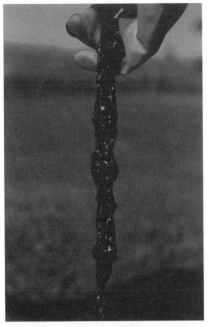

Rubbery Mucoid Plaque Rope

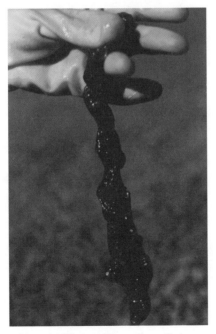

Mucoid Plaque Rope from Colon

Dangers Of Mucoid Plaque

When mucoid accumulations augment, the peristaltic action in the intestines may become less and less effective, and one form or another of constipation or diarrhea often develops. Now I'm sorry to say, most people are constipated. As stated in Chapter 2, **constipation is characterized by having less than two bowel movements daily, and even having two is less than ideal.** A gradual weakening of the body's immune system may also occur after a long-term toxic bowel environment destroys the natural bacterial environment, causes nutritional deficiencies (especially B vitamins and amino acids), weakens the liver, induces congestion, and interferes with nerve meridian points related to hundreds of other parts of our anatomy. **As bowel problems advance, dis-ease conditions also advance, seemingly in direct proportion to the dysfunction of the digestive processes and electrolyte deficiencies.** After all, the bowel – the digestive system – is the hub of our entire body. Every single cell depends upon the digestion of our food. For those who truly care about their health, the following statement should be emphasized and placed at the top of their list of health concepts: **The bowel feeds every organ, every tissue, every cell in our bodies. When the bowel environment and function has become contaminated or inefficient, the cells and organs in the rest of the body will reflect that contamination and dysfunction. A toxic and acid bowel means toxic blood and lymph, toxic organs and cells, and poor health.**

In the words of P.L. Clark, B.S., M.D., Ph.Sa., "Acidosis and toxicosis are the primary causes of all dis-ease. Rid the body of these poisons and correct the habits of living, and good health will be regained and maintained." And, "Just as maggots and flies require the filth of the manure pile in which they grow and propagate, so the human organism must become broken down and filthy through bad habits of living before the tissues and juices of the body will permit the harboring and growth of any noxious bacteria." And he continues, "However, in view of the scientific researchers, whose insights have been cast aside by conventional medicine, it is just as reasonable to assume that the maggots and flies found in a manure pile caused the manure pile, as it is to assume that the various kinds of germs and bacteria, bacilli, or microorganisms, by whatever name you may call them, found in a thoroughly filthy body poisoned with food, drugs, and bad habits caused the condition of ill health." [47]

---

[47] P. L. Clark, B.S., M.D., Ph.Sa., *How to Live and Eat for Health*, 5th edition, (Chicago, IL: The Health School, 1929), pg. 60, 74, 75.

Scientific studies have shown that even a small layer of mucoid plaque appears to **function as a barrier to effective digestion and absorption, and may cause protein and carbohydrate intolerance**. For there are more than 22 known digestive enzymes that are secreted into the intestines, which are essential for thorough digestion. When mucoid plaque lines the intestines, how can these enzymes make contact with the food we hope to digest? And even if there are enough enzymes to digest the food, how can the food be absorbed through the intestinal wall? And poorly digested food is a major contributor to toxicity.

At least 95% of the people who have used our program have found mucoid plaque being eliminated from their bodies, and most of them have improved their health, increased their energy, and eliminated a large spectrum of dis-ease conditions. This indicates that the elimination of the substance called mucoid plaque, and the deep systemic cleansing that occurs with our cleansing program, removes a debilitating level of toxicity and acids closely associated with the loss of vitality and with chronic dis-ease. Countless written testimonies and verbal statements of people have provided strong evidence of the value and validity of intestinal cleansing.

Experienced Doctors on Mucoid Plaque

On page 23 of his book *Tissue Cleansing Through Bowel Management*, Dr. Jensen D.C., N.D., Ph.D. describes mucoid plaque. "The heavy mucus coating in the colon thickens and becomes a host of putrefaction. The blood capillaries to the colon begin to pick up the toxins, poisons and noxious debris as [they seep] through the bowel wall. All tissues and organs of the body are now taking on toxic substances. Here is the beginning of true autointoxication on a physiological level." On page 27, he reveals his knowledge in this matter. **"One autopsy revealed a colon to be 9 inches in diameter with a passage through it no larger than a pencil. The rest was caked up layer upon layer of encrusted fecal material. This accumulation can have the consistency of truck-tire rubber. It's that hard and black.** Another autopsy **revealed a stagnant colon to weigh in at an incredible 40 pounds**. Imagine carrying around all that morbid accumulated waste."

That's astounding, when you stop to consider that the healthy colon should weigh 4 to 6 pounds. This increased weight, especially of the transverse colon, weakens its structure and causes prolapsus, which in turn puts pressure upon the lower organs and weakens them (creating prostate, bladder, and gynecological problems). People who have this augmented profile have what we call "Dunlap Dis-ease," which means *the belly done lapped over the belt*! They are the ones who cannot see their feet when they stand up straight. It is actually a serious condition. I can say confidently that it is only a matter of time and these people will have a life-threatening dis-ease. What's your waistline?

On page 42 of his book, Dr. Jensen talks about his former teacher, Dr. John Harvey Kellogg at the Battle Creek Sanitarium, who maintained that "**90% of the dis-eases of civilization are due to improper functioning of the colon.**" Dr. Jensen explains that National College in Chicago performed over 300 autopsies, and that "according to the history of these persons, 285 had claimed they were not constipated and had normal movements and only 15 had admitted they were constipated. However, autopsies revealed the opposite to be the case, for only 15 were found not to have been constipated, while 285 were found to have been constipated. Some of the histories of these 285 persons stated they had had as many as 5 or 6 bowel movements daily, **yet autopsies revealed that in some of them the bowel was 12 inches in diameter.** The bowel walls were encrusted with material (in one case, peanuts) which had been lodged there for a very long time." Dr. Jensen explains: "As we work with **eliminating the encrusted mucus lining**, we must also consider nourishing the new cells below it.... **Bowel cleansing is an essential element in any lasting healing program. The toxic waste must be removed as quickly as possible to halt the downward spiral of failing health.** This is best done by: 1. **Removing accumulated fecal material from the bowel...**"

Another author, **Dr. Robert Gray**, has described the mucoid plaque in a manner similar to Dr. Jensen's and mine when he states that constipation can be associated with "old, hardened feces" which stick to the walls of the colon and do not pass out with the regular bowel movements. He points out that fecal matter can become sticky and gluey, gluing a coating of itself to the walls of the colon as it passes through. He claims that when "**layer after layer of gluey feces piles up in the colon, they often form into a tough, rubbery black substance.** Old feces may build up in pockets and they may coat the entire length of the colon and small intestines as well. They do not pass from the body with ordinary bowel movements but require special techniques to dissolve the glue, which binds them in the body." Dr. Gray also explains that parasites lodge themselves in the old matter that encrusts the walls of the intestinal tract. He believes that **without the mucoid plaque, intestinal parasites cannot maintain a foothold in the body and to remove the parasites, one must remove the 'mucoid matter.'** He further explains that malabsorption is related to the accumulation of mucoid plaque.[48]

---

[48] Dr. Robert Gray, "The Colon Health Handbook," (Reno. NV: Emerald Publishing, 1986), pg. 5 - 13.

Dr. Jensen and Dr. Gray have different theories from mine as to how the "mucoid plaque" is formed. Both of these authors have stated that it is the acids, toxins, and chemicals in food, especially the highly processed foods that contribute towards the formation of mucoid plaque. I agree that they may contribute towards its composition; however, my studies indicated that excess intake of acid-forming foods drains electrolytes and acidifies the bile which then triggers the mucin to coat the intestines. This is one reason why mucoid plaque forms perfectly to every crease, crack, and fold in the gut.

Dr. V. E. Irons, a pioneer in colon cleansing theory and activity, and a staunch opponent of modern medicine wrote a booklet called: "The Destruction of Your Own Natural Protective Mechanism." In his booklet he made the following statements:

"I challenge the world that you couldn't find in the USA, 1000 people who don't have a clogged colon. Just let me get them on the Colema Board and on the 7-Day Cleansing Program both at the same time and we will show any challengers WHAT WE MEAN. We will let them see, feel and even hold in their hands exactly what has been thickening, hardening, and decaying in their colon for years, causing all types of dis-ease. The conditions of the colons in this entire country are FAR WORSE than either the doctors, the AMA, the drug houses, ... or even the natural health industry have any conception ... and believe in our theory that the CAUSE OF MOST CONDITIONS OF ILL HEALTH IS AUTOINTOXICATION and that 95% of their troubles start in the colon.

We can prove that we can find hardened mucous with its foul smelling curd in the colons of 95% of the entire nation. HOW DO WE KNOW THIS? Because possibly 99% of all ages and sexes have violated two of the major Natural Laws from one to three times every day since they were 2 years old. What are the two laws? 1. The WRONG combination of foods. 2. The constant daily use of tremendous amounts of DEAD FOODS. The wrong application of both of these laws has caused the body's natural protective mechanism to secrete mucous into the colon to protect the body from absorbing the many poisons, which those counterfeit foods create.

But we have simply OVERWORKED** Nature's protective mechanism **to the point that the mechanism

*instead of protecting us from poisons now itself poisons us... This protective mechanism was never designed to continue secreting mucus one layer on top of another layer for years with no time out or chance for its elimination. **The result is that layer on top of layer is secreted until its accumulation thickens to 1/8" to 1/4" thick. Sometimes this layer or layers get to 3/8" to 1/2" in thickness, becoming as hard and black as a piece of old hardened rubber you see on a highway from a truck tire.** It cannot be cut with a knife but you can cut it with a razor blade. Usually it breaks into innumerable small pieces. But we have had specimens saved in alcohol from several inches to a few feet in length while the longest we have had was 27 ft. (in one piece). Sometimes it will come out as a pile weighing as much as 11 lbs. ...and continue to come out for several days to a week...before the old hardened accumulated mucus, so tightly imbedded in the colon for months or years, comes out. It has probably been slowly emitting poisons into your blood stream, causing all types of distorted symptoms. Once this hardened mucous starts to eliminate, it will be trapped in the colander so that you can wash it and examine it.*

Anyone who disagrees with any of the above – REMEMBER, you CAN PROVE it to your own satisfaction by what comes from your own body for the smallest conceivable investment. There is no substitute for experience, and we challenge everyone to experience this for themselves...You (meaning the reader and 95% of the USA) DO HAVE THIS HARDENED MUCUS IN YOUR COLON AND YOU WILL BE AMAZED AT WHAT COMES OUT OF YOU."

My experience has undoubtedly verified Dr. Irons' descriptive explanations. However, a few important points should be addressed: 1) Not all mucoid plaque is as hard as a truck tire, but most people will see some that comes close to that description, 2) It isn't always black; although many people report that theirs was black, usually it is blackish green (it may also come out brown, yellow, white, gray or green); and 3) Not everyone has it in them, but my estimation is that close to 99% of the people who have used the Cleanse have removed it.

A certain doctor from Mexico sent me the following letter. I have not received permission to use his name publicly, so I will give you only his credentials: **M.D., Ph.D., N.D., P.P. Gen. Adm.** A relevant portion of his testimony is recorded here:

> *"Dear Sirs: ... Many times when practicing autopsies on people who died from chronic illnesses,* **I have always found a thick layer of organized mucus-like hardened material** *all over from the tongue down to the stomach, small, large and recto-sigmoid colon. Usually* **it is more common among milk drinkers and meat eaters.** *If for some reason your products have the ability to detach this layer of morbus material, then a great deal of accomplishment will be achieved for these persons. This layer is composed of coagulated and racemized glycoproteins, which* **really impair the GI tract function and also constitute a reservoir of bacteria and viruses that invade the lymph and the blood causing a wearing down of the bodily defenses and significant burden on the liver's detoxification function.** *For that reason, Gerson, Kelly and Beard [relied] always on GI tract cleansing* **to obtain better results with their cancer treatments.** *In the past* **we have even removed the entire colon to obtain effective relief from autointoxication,** *especially with colon polyposis and diverticulosis and chronic ulcerative colitis..."*

Doctors of Great Success

In the early 1900's, **Dr. J. H. Tilden** of Denver, Colorado, specialized in healing pneumonia, which was at that time the number-one killer. During that epidemic almost every doctor lost hundreds of patients to that deadly plague. Dr. Bernard Jensen, who studied with Dr. Tilden, has stated that at that time, Dr. Tilden **treated more pneumonia cases than most and he never lost a patient. He used no drugs at all. He simply cleansed the colon** using enemas and colonics, and administered natural, live foods. Even in those days, his success was considered miraculous because other doctors were relying on drugs and continually meeting with failure.

Doctor Bernard Jensen, D.C., N.D., Ph.D., is one of the truly great doctors. In the 1970's he had a 40% success rate in treating leukemia. This was phenomenal when compared to the 0% rate of success for conventional medicine. He was successful with most patients who came to him, and many had been told by their M.D.s that they had an incurable dis-ease. At the age of 90 he cured himself of a so-called "incurable dis-ease." He made the following statement: **"In the 50 years I've spent helping people to overcome illness, disability and dis-ease, it has become crystal clear that poor bowel management lies at the root of most people's health problems.**[49] Dr. Bernard Jensen had studied with many very successful doctors throughout the Untied States and Europe. He then built his own sanitarium and practiced with an open mind for over 50 years. His fame has been acknowledged worldwide; he was even nominated for the Nobel Prize, but because he was not a "mainstream" doctor, his nomination was rejected.

Dr. Jensen says, "Every tissue is fed by the blood, which is supplied by the bowel. When the bowel is dirty, the blood is dirty, and so on to the organs and tissues... it is the bowel that invariably has to be cared for first before any effective healing can take place." Dr. Jensen publicly stated that more than 90% of all dis-ease in America can be traced to unhealthy conditions in the bowel. Privately, he told me that it's closer to 100%.

In his textbook on iridology, Dr. Jensen explains: "Besides these world-renowned exponents of intestinal sanitation, other authorities have given recognition to the belief that cleanliness of the colon is necessary to good health. It is believed that disorders such as appendicitis, infected tonsils, liver and gallbladder infections, dysfunction of the heart and blood vessels, sinusitis, arthritis, and rheumatism, etc., no doubt have their origin in a sluggish colon."

My experience proves that he is absolutely correct, but I would add one thing – it is not just the colon; in fact, even more important is the small intestine. Doctors who have achieved fame for their exceptional health improvement rates always took care of the alimentary canal. Dr. William Koch; Dr. Eugene Blass; Dr. John Kellogg of the Battle Creek Sanitarium, Sir W. Arbuthnot Lane, surgeon for the King of England; Dr. Bernard Jensen; Dr. John Christopher; and Dr. J.H. Tilden are some of the exceptional individuals who used this knowledge. Sir Arbuthnot Lane, M.S., F.R.C.S., surgeon for the King of England, made the following statement, "I am exceedingly impressed by the sequence of cancer and intestinal stasis." He also said, "There is but one dis-ease and that is deficient drainage."[50] And Dr. P. L. Clark, M.D., verified, "Where there is perfect drainage, there is no death."

---

[49] Bernard Jensen, Ph.D., N.D., D.C., M.H., *Tissue Cleansing Through Bowel Management*, (Escondido, CA: Bernard Jensen Publications, 1981), pg. 3.

[50] Stan Malstrom, N.D., M.T., "Your Colon: Its Character, Care and Therapy," (Orem, Utah: BiWorld Publications, Inc., 1981), pg. 1.

Dr. Lane spent many years specializing in bowel problems. He was an expert in removing sections of the bowel and stitching the remainder back together. He taught this work to other doctors and gained an international reputation for his efficiency. During the years of this work, he began to notice a peculiar phenomenon: During the course of recovery from colonic surgery, some of his patients experienced remarkable cures of dis-eases that had no apparent connection with his surgery. For instance, a young boy who had had arthritis for many years, and was in a wheelchair at the time of surgery, recovered entirely from his arthritis six months after his surgery. Another case involved a woman with a goiter. When a specific section of the bowel was removed in surgery, there ensued a definite remission of the goiter within six months.

These and similar experiences impressed Dr. Lane deeply, as he saw the relationship between the toxic bowel and the functioning of various organs in the body. After much thought about this relationship, he became very interested in changing the bowel through dietetic methods and spent the last 25 years of his life teaching people how to care for the bowel through cleansing and nutrition, and not surgery. Referring to a toxic bowel, he wrote, "The poisons thus generated pollute the bloodstream, causing every tissue, gland, and organ of the body to gradually deteriorate and be destroyed." Lane also stated that, 1.) "Arthritis could not develop in the absence of intestinal toxemia; 2.) There is clinical and x-ray evidence of stasis in such patients; and, 3.) The symptoms disappear and patients recover sometimes with startling rapidity when the condition of stasis has been effectively [handled]." Lane reports a connection between intestinal toxemia and "several changes in the thyroid," such as "adenomatous growths." He also made this statement to the staff of John Hopkins Hospital and Medical College: "Gentlemen, I will never die of cancer. I am taking measures to prevent it. It is caused by poisons created in our bodies by the food we eat...."

Dr. Harvey Kellogg, M.D., of the Kellogg Sanitarium, said, "Of the 22,000 operations that I have personally performed, I have never found a single normal colon, and of the 100,000 that were performed under my jurisdiction, not over 6% were normal."[51] Dr. Kellogg said that he knew of many cases in which operations were prevented by cleansing and revitalizing the bowel. He maintained that 90% of the dis-eases of civilization are due to improper functioning of the colon.

---

[51] Bernard Jensen, Ph.D., N.D., D.C., *Iridology: The Science and Practice in the Healing Arts*, Volume II, (Escondido, CA: Bernard Jensen Publications, 1982), pg. 408.

Dr. George C. Crile, head of the Crile Clinic in Cleveland and one of the world's greatest surgeons, said, "There is no natural death. All deaths that come from so-called natural causes are merely the end point of progressive acid saturation. Many people go so far as to consider that sickness and dis-ease are just a 'cross' or an element, which God gave them to bear here on this earth. However, if they would take care of their bodies and cleanse the colon and intestines, their problems would be pretty much eliminated and they could eliminate their 'cross' by proper diet, proper exercise, and in general, proper living."

Many doctors have proven that the bowel is the key to health or dis-ease and the most important part of our physical anatomy to take care of in order to achieve successful healing. Most of the following cases were obtained from medical journals printed before 1930. You see, this information had been known, acknowledged, and taught. But its use would decrease potential medical and drug profits. If the medical monopoly was to become a multi-trillion-dollar-a-year industry, the knowledge about bowel cleansing and fasting had to be suppressed and denied.

William Lintz, M.D., successfully treated 472 patients suffering from allergies by cleansing the bowel. Allan Eustis, M.D., Professor at Tulane University of Medicine in 1912, cured 121 cases of bronchial asthma by intestinal cleansing. D. Rochester, M.D., University of Buffalo School of Medicine in 1906, made the statement that after 23 years of observation, he concluded that toxemia of gastrointestinal tract origin is the underlying cause of asthma. Dr. Bassler reported that by reducing intestinal toxemia, he had 100% success eliminating cardiac arrhythmia. Dr. Bainbridge (M.D.), stated that intestinal toxemia is common among the causative factors of so-called functional heart dis-ease. Dr. D. J. Barry stated, "There seems little doubt that substances having a deleterious action on the heart musculature and nerves, are formed both in the small and large intestine, even under apparently normal circumstances." Dr. Hovel stated that "toxemia due to intestinal sepsis is a common cause of increased blood pressure." J. A. Stucky, M.D.: "In several hundreds of cases of dis-eases of the nasal accessory sinuses, middle and internal ear... I have found unmistakable and marked evidence of toxemia of intestinal origin as evidenced by excessive indican in the urine, and when the condition causing this was removed there was marked amelioration or entire relief of the dis-ease." C. W. Hawley, M.D., treated many cases of eyestrain and dis-ease with success once again by relieving intestinal toxemia. In 1892, a Dr. Herter (M.D.) linked intestinal putrefaction to epilepsy in 31 patients.

One doctor who used our Cleanse had epilepsy. During her cleanse she had her last seizure. Five years later she reported that she has never had a seizure since doing our Cleanse and has had no other signs of epilepsy.

Research involving autism has found that seizures may be associated with certain toxic bacteria.[52] It appears that when these bacteria are present in certain individuals, seizures can occur. The Cleanse is obviously one of the most effective methods of reducing large amounts of bacteria very quickly. This could be a problem for those rare individuals who have that type of bacteria that produces epilepsy, when they use a powerful cleansing program. Deep cleansing could stir up these little buggers, which could possibly activate a seizure. As indicated above, this has occurred, but fortunately, as also indicated, it may be the last one. It is impossible to know for certain. But, if I had epilepsy, guess what I would do?

Drs. Satterlee and Eldridge reported their experience with 518 cases of "mental symptoms," including "mental sluggishness, dullness, and stupidity; loss of concentration and/or memory; mental incoordination, irritability, lack of confidence, excessive and useless worry." Their success in eliminating these symptoms by surgically relieving intestinal toxemia is truly remarkable in the light of today's commonly held beliefs. When people remove the toxicity and congestion that interfere with mental problems, they can expect improvement. And this is common while cleansing.

When my mother reached the age of 81 she began to "lose it," as they say. My sister had called me to warn me that when I visited mother I should be prepared, for she could hardly remember what she had done or said just five minutes earlier. Sure enough, I was shocked, for she had always had an almost perfect memory. And talk? She never stopped, but the worst thing of all was that she would constantly repeat herself about every five minutes. It was disgusting. Finally, I convinced her to do a Cleanse. In fact I redesigned it, making it the easiest and mildest cleanse ever! Even though it was the Mildest Phase and she was only on it for two and one-half weeks, she had marvelous results. Not only did her memory return, but it was better than ever. She could remember just about every detail of her life from when she was a little child up to the present. And now, at 87 years of age, she is alert as ever.

---

[52] See "Autism and Microorganisms," Videotape Series: Tape 1, William Shaw, Ph.D., Great Plains Laboratory, Overland Park, KS. Phone 913-341-8949. Dr. Shaw explains that bacteria and yeast produce certain specific compounds, which are absorbed into the blood and eventually secreted into the urine. New sensitive equipment are now able to measure these compounds. It has been found that bowel toxins are far more prevalent than once thought. Dr. Shaw associates bowel toxins with Rett's syndrome, seizures, adult and child psychoses, severe depression, attention deficit, hyperactivity, and hypoglycemia. A little more research, and they may find much more than that.

Dr. J. F. Burgess, Montreal General Hospital, reported the results of studying 109 cases of eczema. He states, "On the basis of clinical observations and sensitivity tests against various amino acids and ptomaine bases, eczema is probably caused by intestinal toxemia." A few years ago a nurse, who had endured horrible eczema for over 30 years, did the Cleanse. Of course most of the doctors whom she had worked with had prescribed one kind of drug after another, with no lasting results. After one Cleanse, more than 90% of her eczema disappeared.

All dis-ease is an internal environmental mutation. It is my own opinion that all cancer, AIDS, disorders of the liver, kidney, brain, and heart receive their mutating potential, in the form of toxins and congestion, from the intestines. And when this mutating potential is not directly associated with the bowel, then it is because the liver, kidneys, or other organs have become weakened as a result of long-term bowel toxicity. Other factors are nutrient deficient foods, negative thoughts, etc., each of which affect the bowel. Sir Arbuthnot Lane tried to make it clear when he wrote that he was "exceedingly impressed by the sequence of cancer and intestinal stasis."

Mucoid Plaque, Toxins, Acids, and Free Radicals

When the intestines contain mucoid plaque, an interference with the digestive process results. An inefficient digestive system will cause some degree of malnutrition and toxicity because food is not thoroughly digested, nor absorbed.

Mucoid plaque may contribute towards fermentation, putrefaction (rotting), and stagnant pus pockets holding various poisons and harmful bacteria or parasites in the bowel. Clinical studies have shown that pathogenic bacteria, particularly *E. coli*, can pass through a mucoid layer in less than 2 hours and be completely separated and protected from luminal contents. The mucoid plaque serves as a stronghold and protects the pathogen from whatever luminal[53] attack a doctor may wish to administer. *E. Coli*, by the way, is one of the pathogenic bacteria that is known to stimulate mucoid plaque secretion.

Sometimes pockets of pus and debris settle and accumulate to such a degree that the colon's circumference expands to four or more times its

---

[53] "Luminal" (adj.) or "lumen" (n.) refers to the passageway of the intestines, the route our food takes – a corridor, like the hole in a donut.

normal size. Is it any wonder most people have bulging lower abdomens and "Dunlap Dis-ease?"

Commonly, smaller pockets start protruding beyond the colon wall, forming diverticulitis. This is the most perfect internal environment for worms, parasites, and pathogenic bacteria. It is in these areas that colon cancer often develops. You didn't really think that cancer just appears without cause, did you?

These toxins and poisons cause excessive acids and stress upon our bodies. The stress plus nutritional deficiencies allow free radicals to be generated far beyond healthy proportions. Free radicals are associated with heart dis-ease, cancer, Alzheimer's disease, Parkinson's disease, rheumatoid arthritis, premature aging, etc.[54]

It should be increasingly clear that toxicity in our bodies is an extreme and potentially deadly disadvantage. Whatever area in the body accumulates toxins also becomes weak, sluggish, tired, and ineffective. And weak areas give way to ever-increasing toxic overloads, which is where dis-ease develops. As one health expert put it, **"The name of a dis-ease depends upon where the poisons settle.** Thus, from the same source, various names of dis-ease are given."** Even if one succeeds in strengthening the weak area or suppressing the symptom, the toxic flow from the bowel will find another area to break through. **Dis-ease can only permanently be overcome when the cause is remedied. And removing cause includes removing toxins and congestion.**

Dis-ease is a Creation – The Remedy is Obvious

It should be increasingly clear to you, the reader, that dis-ease is a natural by-product of an unnatural lifestyle. Can you see now that it is the unnatural things we do to ourselves that forces the body into one situation after another until it loses its ability to maintain natural balance? In *Cleanse & Purify Thyself*, Book 2, I make it even clearer. In that book you

---

[54] A free radical is a molecule that has lost one of its electrons and becomes hungry for another one. After a free radical has lost one of its electrons, it becomes dangerous to other molecules because it can steal one of their electrons. It is like someone who was bit by a vampire and became a vampire himself. Once a molecule becomes imbalanced in this way, it damages cells. It can create a chain reaction and cause a chain reaction of cell damage and premature aging. Antioxidants are needed to stop this terrible destruction.

can learn the chemical process with which we create our own dis-ease. In my book *UnCreating Dis-ease*, it becomes even clearer. Dis-ease, you see, is a creation, not an accident. We do not acquire dis-ease; we do not get germs or catch colds "just because." We must first weaken our immune system before we can "catch" something. We cannot "catch" a germ – a bacteria, yeast, or parasite – until after we have created the right circumstances and environment for its propagation. It is the milieu that makes the difference – *c'est le mileu qui compte*. We must create the dis-ease environment before we can have a dis-ease.

Every life-form on the planet survives in a specific environment. **Change the environment and you automatically change the species that reside in that habitat**. As you will never see a giraffe in the Arctic, nor a penguin in the tropics, you will also never see normal friendly microorganisms in an acid bowel. Nor will we see pathogenic bacteria, yeast, or parasites in a clean, healthy body.

And to reverse dis-ease conditions, **we must first stop doing everything we had been doing which caused this dis-ease condition to develop in the first place**. We must also **remove everything in our bodies that creates a malfunction**. Now, that seems logical to me; I hope it is logical to you, but this logic has been lost and, surprisingly, most doctors can't see it, for if they did, they would change their ways. So remember this very important statement: **Whatever we have put into the body that interferes with its ability to function properly must be removed**. And that includes toxins, poisons, industrial chemicals, heavy metals, pathogenic microorganisms, parasites, etc., etc. Truly think about it, and then Cleanse & Purify Thyself.

Now you can see that even if you eat the most perfect foods, you may still have problems. **Eating the most perfect foods is no guarantee that you will assimilate and use the nutrients your body requires**. It is no guarantee that perfect food will not ferment and rot in your body. For, if your body cannot digest food properly, you will have trouble.

If you understand this chapter, you know more about the cause of dis-ease and its proper treatment than the entire medical system demonstrates. For if the medical world would try to understand these simple truths and learn to treat the cause of dis-ease with Nature's perfect methods designed for man by God – instead of relying on drugs, radiation and scalpels designed by man – their continual failures would become successes. Though this would not enhance their pocketbooks, the planet would become a world of healthy, happy, and prosperous people.

I was talking about treating causes with a fellow once who insisted, "When I get a flat tire, I just fix it. I don't worry about causes." I replied, "Would you try to fix the leaking hole in the tire while the nail was still in it?" He said, "Oh. I see your point." Doctors do the very same thing when they cut out cancer in a colon or breast. They leave the cause. Patients go home and pray that it doesn't come back again. Seldom are they told to change their diets. They are rarely given nutritional advice. And they are never told to clean out the toxicity and filth that is causing their suffering. They go home and keep on doing what they did that created their problems in the first place. They are told to "enjoy life," *if* they can.

You may be wondering about chemotherapy and radiation therapy – will those treatments remove the cause? Emphatically, no! They even contribute towards it. Radiation therapy damages the esophagus, intestinal mucosa, and the liver. It can cause liver toxicity: It has affected up to 50% of patients exposed to total-body **irradiation and chemotherapy, and has led to liver failure in one-third (1/3) of patients affected.**[55] And liver failure, I might add, means death. Chemotherapy has caused toxicity in over 80% of the patients and inflicts serious damage to the liver, bile ducts, stomach, and duodenum.[56] These harsh treatments significantly increase toxicity and weaken the body terribly. After such severe treatments, the entire body's immune system is essentially destroyed. And did you know that cancer cannot live in a body with a strong immune system? **Does it make sense to you for doctors to destroy the immune system when the immune system is needed to destroy the cancer? Why don't they build the immune system instead of destroying it?** Such treatments are never the better part of wisdom; they're foolish beyond reason. Truly we live in a medical dark age. For information on this subject, I suggest my book *UnCreating Dis-ease.*[57]

---

[55] Yamada, pg. 903.

[56] Ibid., pg. 1804.

[57] Anderson, *UnCreating Dis-ease*. Read the entire story to learn how disease is created and "un-created." Cancer – its cause and treatment – is also addressed; why conventional cancer treatments do not work, and actually create harm and death. It also covers how viruses, bacteria, yeasts, and other microorganisms are created within our own bodies, how the mind controls physiological functions, and more.

CHAPTER 4

UNVEILED MYSTERIES OF HEALTH AND HEALING

"As all creatures come forth from the unseen into this world, so they return to the unseen, and so will they come again 'til they be purified."[58]

– Jesus of Nazareth

"Mind doesn't dominate body, it becomes body – body and mind are one."

– Candace B. Pert, Ph.D.

I have studied health and the mind now for over 37 years, and I can say that the most important factor in health, longevity, and overcoming dis-ease is attitude – our daily points of view. This is covered with more detail in my books *Cleanse & Purify Thyself,* Book 2, and *UnCreating Dis-ease.* For it is our attitudes that govern our eating habits, our digestion and assimilation of food, our lifestyles, our glandular and immune systems, and even the function of every cell in our bodies.

Thoughts and Feelings – The Primal Causes of Health or Dis-ease

Experience has taught me, as noted above, that the real causes of dis-ease are the negative attitudes we promote with misguided thoughts and feelings to which we consciously or unconsciously devote our energy. We live in a universe that is ruled by exact law, and being ignorant of it does not exclude its effect upon us. Truly, for every action there is a reaction. Isaac Newton was certainly not the first who taught this law; Buddha and,

---

[58] *The Gospel of the Perfect Life*, 94:2, (Mt. Shasta, CA: Christobe Publishing, projected publication 2001).

later Jesus Christ, and thousands of others beat him to it. I wonder why he received all the credit. And, how does this law apply here? Our thoughts and feelings are potent forces of energy and vibration and help direct and manifest specific conditions in our lives. **They control all cells in our bodies, and they even control DNA.** More than any other factor, thoughts and feelings **create our lives as they are today and as they will be tomorrow and every other tomorrow.** In my opinion, every single thing in existence is a creation associated with thoughts and feelings. The greatest of all philosophers and spiritual leaders agreed with this concept and now, at last, science is proving it. Today there are volumes of medical journals and thousands of studies that support this theory. [59]

Understanding this theory is one thing, dealing with the emotions is another. I have been researching this subject since 1964 and have made some important discoveries. For an example I have seen people struggle with certain issues for decades and in the space of only *one (1!)* cleanse I have seen them release a primary issue and have it never return. I wanted to know the reasons and to some degree, I have found them.

Here are a few observations my study has revealed[60]:

- ❑ Emotions get trapped in cells and when we fast or cleanse, these emotion-carrying cells, especially the weak, dead, or dying cells are rapidly released from the body. In this way we release forever the emotions that were trapped in those cells.
- ❑ Emotions and intelligence can be transmitted from one cell to another. But when holding a positive attitude while cleansing, we prevent the cells from transmitting their emotions to another cell.
- ❑ More emotions are stored in the mucoid plaque than most other parts of our bodies.
- ❑ When we cleanse or fast, striking emotional transformation often occurs when mucoid plaque is released.

An old Chinese axiom; found in the I Ching, states, "That which is above is as that which is below, and that which is below is as that which is above." If this is a universal truth, then it should be evident that the body reflects the mind, and impurities of either are reflected in the other.

Just as sound in its own octave contains enough solidity to impress our ear drums to hear, and light is substantial enough to impress upon our

---

[59] For scientific verification that the primal causes of dis-ease are our thoughts and feelings, read *Molecules of Emotion: The Science Behind Mind-Body Medicine*, by Candace B. Pert, Ph.D. (New York, NY: Touchstone, 1999).

[60] As noted on page 20, the "box bullets" indicate informational points.

retina to see, so thoughts and feelings are also real and substantial enough to exert powerful effects upon our consciousness and bodies. Thoughts and feelings not only stimulate and control our glandular systems and influence all the cells in our bodies, but they also **solidify into our bodies and minds in a way that either brings forth congestion or circulation – good health or dis-ease**.

Mind is the Master Power
that molds and makes
And man is mind
and forevermore he takes
his tools of thought
and shaping what he wills
brings forth a thousand joys,
a thousand ills.
He thinks in secret,
and it comes to pass.
Environment
is but his looking glass.

- Ella Wheeler Wilcox

I am attempting to impress upon the minds of my readers that the mind is truly the key to health and to dis-ease. It is always a distortion of the mind that causes people to commit harmful acts against themselves and others. Smoking, using drugs, and becoming intoxicated from drinking alcohol are obvious examples. As I said, the way we eat is also controlled by the mind via the subconscious mind, and we may suffer according to foolish and uncontrolled desires. People should be asking themselves how they became the way they are; how they created their problems. Seek within. Look for the cause with no blame or guilt. And as we inquire from within, we soon realize that we are indeed subject to certain universal laws, which Newton described in acceptable terms.

Consider the words of the Master Jesus, whose well-known sayings include the following: "Ye shall pay even the last penny"; and "That which you sow shall you also reap"; and "According to your faith it is done unto you." Most of us are affected by the past more than the Now. Thoughts and feelings of the past constantly exude into our brains, bodies and environments, producing the cause behind the cause. Man may be unjust, but Nature (God) is not. If we are not satisfied with our minds, bodies, and conditions in our lives, as they are, we must "cleanse and purify" and "sin no more." I am about to quote from *The Gospel of Peace of Jesus Christ* by the disciple John, which is one of the most interesting books about health that I have ever read. It is full of wisdom and truth. My comments are in italics and brackets, and boldface treatment is mine, for emphasis. After reading this you may think that it is a prophecy of the 20th and 21st century. [61]

*"I tell you, **unless you follow the laws of your Mother, you can in no wise escape death**. And he who clings to the laws of his Mother, to him shall his Mother cling also. [Perhaps we should take better care of Mother Earth.] She shall heal all his plagues, and he shall never become sick. She gives him long life, and protects him from all afflictions; from fire, from water, from the bite of venomous serpents. For your Mother who bore you, keeps life within you. She has given you her body, **and none but she heals you**. Happy is he who loves his Mother and lies quietly in her bosom. For, your Mother loves you, even when you turn away from her. And how much more shall she love you, if you turn to her again? I tell you truly, very great is her love, greater than the greatest of mountains, deeper than the deepest seas. And those who love their Mother, she never deserts them. As the hen protects her chickens, as the lioness her cubs, as the mother her newborn babe, so does the Earthly Mother protect the son of Man from all danger and from all evils.*

*For I tell you truly, evils and dangers innumerable lie in wait for the Sons of Men. Beelzebub, the prince of all devils, the source of every evil, lies in wait in the body of all the Sons of Men. [Could this be the human ego - the source of discordant thoughts, feelings and destructive desires?] He is death, the lord of every plague, **and taking upon him a pleasing raiment**, [which may be hamburgers and coke] **he tempts and entices the Sons of Men**. Riches does he promise, and power, and splendid palaces, and garments of gold and silver, and a multitude of servants, all these; he promises renowned glory, fornication and lustfulness, gluttony and wine-bibbing, riotous living, and slothfulness and idle days.*

***And he entices every one by that to which their heart is most inclined**. [Ouch, that hurt!] And in the day that the Sons of Men have already become the slaves of all these vanities and abominations [slaves to our own*

---

[61] The American version is titled *The Essene Gospel of Peace*, edited by Edmond Bordeaux Szekely.

thoughts, lusts, desires, appetites, fears, self-pity, resentments, hates, and other habits], *then in payment thereof he snatches from the Sons of Men all those things, which the Earthly Mother gave them so abundantly. He takes from them their breath,* [smokers beware], *their blood,* [cancer, leukemia and other blood disorders], *their bone,* [arthritis and osteoporosis], *their flesh,* [eczema, rashes, leprosy], *their bowels,* [ulcers, constipation, colitis, and cancer of the bowels, etc.], *their eyes and their ears* [Know anyone who wears glasses or hearing aids ? is blind or deaf?].

And the breath of the Son of Man becomes short and stifled, full of pain and evil-smelling, like the breath of unclean beasts [What is your breath like in the morning? Use mouthwash? How far can you run without getting out of breath?]. *And his blood becomes thick and evil smelling, like the water of the swamps; it clots and blackens, like the night of death. And his bone becomes hard and knotted* [arthritis]; *it melts away within and breaks asunder, as a stone falling down upon a rock* [osteoporosis]. *And his flesh waxes fat and watery* [who's overweight in America?]; *it rots and putrefies, with scabs and boils that are an abomination.* **And his bowels become full with abominable filthiness, with oozing streams of decay; and multitudes of abominable worms having their habitation there** [And they knew about it way back then. Think about it! Why haven't medical doctors learned about this yet?].

And his eyes grow dim, till dark night enshrouds them, and his ears become stopped, like the silence of the grave [And even in the 20th and 21st centuries, two-year-old children suffer from stopped-up ears due to use of pasteurized dairy products]. *And last of all shall the erring Son of Man lose life. For, he kept not the laws of his Mother, and added sin to sin. Therefore, are taken from him all the gifts of the Earthly Mother: breath, blood, bone, flesh, bowels, eyes and ears, and after all else, life, with which the Earthly Mother crowned his body* (Truly, this must have been a prophecy of the 20th century).

But if the erring son of Man be sorry for his sins and undo them [to undo them is to cleanse and purify the thoughts, emotions, habits, and our bodies], *and return again to his Earthly Mother; and if he do his Earthly Mother's laws and free himself from Satan's clutches [that human ego again?], resisting his temptation, then does the Earthly Mother receive again her erring Son with love and sends him her angels that they may serve him. I tell you truly, when the Son of Man resists the Satan that dwells in him and does not his will, in the same hour are found the mother's angels there, that they may serve him with all their power and free utterly the Son of Man from the power of Satan.* [Could it be that "Satan" refers to mankind's misuse of his/her creative power of thoughts and feelings? And that the "Mother's angels" are the healthy use of mankind's creative power of thoughts and feelings? Whether it is symbolic as I have suggested, or actual evil and Divine beings, matters little to my way of thinking. The results would be the same].

For no man can serve two masters. For either he serves Beelzebub and his devils, or else he serves our Earthly Mother and her angels. Either he serves death or he serves life. I tell you truly, **happy are those who do the laws of life and wander not upon the paths of death. For in them the forces of life wax strong and they escape the plagues of death."**

The Way Out

From a spiritual viewpoint, our bodies are supposed to be the temples of the Living God. Instead the majority of American bodies have become filled with "abominable filthiness, with oozing streams of decay, and with multitudes of abominable worms having their habitation there." In other words, they have become "seething, smelly cesspools that house fermenting, putrefying, rotting death." And this, my friends, is a scientific fact! We could call it "the Standard American Bowel." There are two main causes - the unnatural and dead foods we have consumed and the inharmonious thoughts and feelings that, sooner or later, solidify physically in the cells and organs of their creator, causing a lack of vital energy and circulation, and dysfunction of cells and organs.

Consistently, we have found that in each locality of weakness or dis-ease, whether it is in an organ, muscle, bone, or whatever, there will also be stored memories of inharmonious thoughts and feelings, which constantly radiate an analogous vibrational message to other cells, molecules, and even DNA. In this manner, intense emotions can modify cell function and mutate DNA, thereby altering the original archetypal blueprint of health. Remove the "stuck" thoughts and feelings, and the toxins move out quickly, the pain dissipates, and circulation, strength, and normal function are reestablished. You may prove this to yourself as you cleanse. For the deeper you cleanse, the more memories, thoughts, feelings, desires, tastes, and smells from the past are recalled. Some memories will return vivid and clear, even though you had, seemingly, totally forgotten them. And here lies the great key to health and longevity. Did you notice? Do you now realize why it behooves you and everyone else who seeks perfect health to "Cleanse & Purify"? And, I should add, to stop producing any feeling that is less than joy, peace, and love. We can do it!

Mucoid Plaque, Protein, and Cells Bind Memories of Emotions and Perpetuate Habits

Most Americans have mucoid plaque and other protein-like substances in their intestines that have been there since they were children and, in some cases, since they were babies. As the old mucoid plaque breaks apart, many people recall and feel incidents that occurred many years ago. These recollections appear to be the same feelings, and are certainly analogous to experiences many years past – possibly when they had been consuming the food that became the mucilage protein composing the mucoid plaque. This is a common experience and has led me to hypothesize that as long **as the protein matter – which contains those old emotions, thoughts, or desires – remains within us, antagonistic memories continue to emit destructive vibrations, and we will continue to be unconsciously influenced by them.** However, once we completed the task of removing protein matter from the bowel, we are then in a position to remove the stuck thoughts and feelings from the rest of our being. And each time we remove another dark or negative thought-form entity, we raise ourselves to another step.

Unresolved Negative Thoughts and Feelings Cause Dis-ease and Limitation

Unresolved emotions have a profound effect upon us. They influence every system and metabolic activity in our bodies – the mind, heart, immunity, glands, muscles, etc. For an example, repressed anger, fear, and despair constrict blood flow and nutrients to the frontal cortex and other organs. The results are limitation in mental function, such as memory, clarity, and concentration, as well as other functions related to the frontal cortex. Unfortunately, with over one hundred years of psychological research, little is known about how to eliminate the negative, unresolved thoughts and emotions that may be causing serious dis-ease. However, I have found that by cleansing the body, we automatically reveal and release suppressed emotions. This is incredibly important for anyone suffering from dis-ease, and for those on a sincere spiritual path. Once this knowledge is fully understood and brought into mainstream medicine, the medical system, as we now know it, will change dramatically and beneficially. Truly, the medicine of the future will deal more with the mind than with drugs. As this understanding advances, we shall also find that social behavior will change and dis-ease will begin to disappear along with war, poverty, and unhappiness. Indeed, one of the greatest needs in this world is for people to realize how their minds control their lives and how to use this information advantageously.

Of the various emotional binding substances within us, the mucoid plaque is, by far, the easiest to extract. Remember, the bowel is the hub of the body, on which the whole body relies, and **after we have cleansed the plaque from the bowel, it becomes within our reach to extract toxicity, mucus, and unresolved conflicts from the rest of our bodies**. Once complete purification has been obtained, and that includes the removal of all inharmonious thoughts and feelings, then the potential of becoming "super-human" beings may also come within our grasp. **For, the emotions of unresolved conflicts most definitely block our fullest potential. Being completely free of inharmonious emotions opens us up to unlimited love, wisdom, ability, and happiness.**

You can prove for yourself this theory that emotions are related to the cause of dis-ease. While cleansing, observe carefully the old memories, thoughts, feelings, desires, tastes, and smells as they arise from the depths of your subconscious. Memories and pictures may come back with vivid clarity even though you thought that you had totally forgotten them. **If you begin feeling unexpected fears, angers, resentment, etc., you will be experiencing some of your causes of dis-ease**. Whether it's a dis-ease that exists now or one that will be in the future matters not; it needs to be transformed. When old experiences arise while cleansing, trace them to the source. Many of them may be the actual feelings that have been the primal cause of a specific dis-ease that has concerned you. Should this happen, rejoice! And visualize yourself in perfect health and happiness and, most important, see yourself as a loving and forgiving person. During these times, however, you may find it difficult to maintain a positive balance, **but if your *intent* is strong enough, it will carry you through**. Fortunately, while cleansing, these emotions and memories are temporary. As soon as the mucoid plaque, proteins, or cells that contain those bits of memory-consciousness are released from the body, they vanish immediately and forever.

Several years ago, a couple came to see me; the woman had a life-threatening cancer. As often happened in the presence of people with cancer, I acquired a severe headache. I stopped our conversation and explained that I had acquired a severe headache, and that the reason was the intensely dark, inharmonious feelings held by the person who had developed the cancer. After a more detailed explanation, I proceeded to show them how we could work together to remove this frightful and destructive thought-form. I told them to ask for assistance from the highest Divine Intelligence they could imagine and then visualize themselves enveloped in blazing, bluish-white Divine Light. "You do this," I said, "and I will do the rest." Within a few seconds we all felt a profound change. Tears of joy flooded everyone in the room. For the next 5 or 10 minutes these two people released a flood of long-suppressed emotions.

After they went home, they began cleansing. More emotions surfaced. A little over a month passed by, and when they came back to see me they informed me that the cancer was completely gone and along with it, all the fear, anger, and worry that the woman had held for several years. Her husband again broke down in tears of deepest gratitude. He then told me that it wasn't just her cancer that had caused such grave concern, but that she also had symptoms indicating that she had been in the process of losing her mind. During the last few years she had been gradually becoming more and more mentally dysfunctional to the point of acute schizophrenia, and she had lost her capacity to consistently think coherently, hold a job, or even drive a car. But all that had vanished the very moment of the exhilaration she experienced while in my office.

Over the years I have seen and heard of hundreds of these kinds of restorations. I have concluded that this, though less dramatic, is actually rather common for those who have used my cleansing program. It doesn't happen with everyone, of course. It seems to occur with those who are ready, whose intent to heal is strong and sincere, who can set aside their denials and scrutinize themselves carefully, and, of course, who follow the directions carefully.

By the late 1980's I had acquired enough experience to realize that the dark feelings I am talking about somehow become trapped in our cells and proteins. I found that when people had their greatest breakthroughs, mucoid plaque – a protein substance – was almost always being released at the exact time as the emotions surfaced. Fortunately, once the mucoid plaque was flushed down the porcelain throne, the emotions vanished forever.

After cleansing for so many years, the mucoid plaque finally stopped coming out me. It appeared that I was free. However, occasionally I would once again be faced with inharmonious emotions, and during those periods I found that by cleansing, fasting, or taking herbal coffee enemas, I shortened the emotional crisis with miraculous speed. During these times, I often found more mucoid plaque once again coming out of my body – not very much, maybe only a few inches. This has been consistent for many years.

Finally, there came a time when I never saw mucoid plaque coming from my body, even while using the full regime of our Cleanse. I then focused upon liver cleansing and probably used almost a hundred different combinations of liver cleansing aids. During this time, I experienced even more unwanted emotions rise within me. Fortunately, I knew what to do, and have since achieved wonderful states of being.

These concepts about thoughts and feelings clinging to the physical body seem aberrant to many; I have always been surprised and delighted that so many doctors hold similar convictions. Most of them, however, are unaware of the connection between mucoid plaque and emotions. For many years I have wished that I could conduct clinical studies to verify these important findings, but a lack of funds has thus far prevented this.

Though many doctors have been aware of the mind-body connection, few have realized its full significance. For years I had searched for scientific verification that our minds and feelings control every function of our bodies. Imagine my joy when one of my colleagues told me about a book that supported, from the highest level of science, what I had been teaching for the past 12 years. I purchased the book, entitled *Molecules of Emotions,* by Candace Pert, Ph.D.[62] She had been doing research in the National Institute of Health, which is the United States government's premier biomedical research establishment. In her book she explains that emotions link mind and body and that emotions run every system in our bodies. She clearly expresses that **repressed emotions are stored in the body at the cellular level** and that "virtually all illness, if not psychosomatic in foundation, has a definite psychosomatic component." She explains how the **"molecules of emotion run every system in our body."** She points out that the body and mind are not separate, and **we**

---

[62] Candace B. Pert, Ph.D., *Molecules of Emotion: The Science Behind Mind-Body Medicine*, (New York, NY: Touchstone, 1999). Dr. Pert is a research professor in the Department of Physiology and Biophysics at Georgetown University Medical Center in Washington D.C.

cannot treat one without the other, and that **the body can and must be healed through the mind**, and that **the mind can and must be healed through the body.**

Very few doctors have realized how thoughts and emotions are stored in the body and actually control every system and function, even the immune system. Even fewer have learned how to extract the emotions that produce dis-ease in our bodies. This is a field new to the world, and one that I have focused upon for many years. In several cases I have seen almost instantaneous healings simply by removing stuck emotions from the body. My experiences have clearly revealed that unresolved emotions are the root cause of most, if not all, dis-ease and that becoming totally free of the unresolved emotions and inharmonious thoughts may produce extraordinary health, longevity, and happiness. These concepts also explain why one medicine will work for one person and not another, for consciousness, not chemistry, produces the final outcome. Its implications on a spiritual level are endless; as Jesus said, "Harken unto me therefore, not only unclean things entering into the body of man defile the man, but much more do evil thoughts and unclean, which pour from the heart of man, defile the inner man and defile others also. Therefore take heed to your thoughts and cleanse your hearts and let your food be pure."[63]

---

[63] *The Gospel of the Perfect Life*, 43:14.

The Gospel of the Perfect Life is also known as the Gospel of the Holy Twelve. It is considered the most accurate and authentic New Testament available. There is little question that the Bible used by orthodox Christianity has been altered to meet the designs of those who wished to control the Christian movement. There is evidence that the *Gospel of the Perfect Life* was used by Saint Francis, who read from it each morning and evening. Compared to the modern New Testament, it is highly inspiring and uplifting. It is full of powerful suggestions to encourage one towards love and responsibility. Jesus had predicated that His words would be altered and misused. He said: "But there shall arise after you, men of perverse minds who shall through ignorance or through craft, suppress many things which I have spoken unto you, and lay to me things which I never taught, sowing tares among the good wheat, which I have given you to sow in the world." (*The Gospel of the Perfect Life,* 44:7.) Various church fathers knew of this particular manuscript of Jesus' life, for it is mentioned various times throughout history, but the manuscript managed to disappear and reappear over and over. Indeed, this book is obviously a serious threat to those who wish to control and manipulate mankind, especially orthodox Christianity. This book has been available to the public for over 100 years, yet it is only known by a few. Other ancient manuscripts about the life and sayings of Jesus have also been kept from the public. The Nag Hammadi manuscripts found in Egypt in 1945, the *Dead Sea Scrolls* discovered in an ancient Essene community called Khirbet Qumran in 1947, and the Gospel of Jesus Christ series still in the Vatican. Why are they hiding the manuscripts? What are they afraid of? Seek and ye shall find out.

In terms of achieving my personal goals of unconditional love and joy, and non-judgment, I have found that in the last two years I have made more progress than in the last 30 years. Why? Because of the releasing of so many unconscious conflicts within myself and because of the work I have been doing with my liver. For, the liver seems to be a doorway into our storehouse of emotions. If you wish for more information on these subjects, read my book *Cleanse & Purify Thyself,* Book 2 and my booklet "The Liver, Cleansing and Rejuvenating The Vital Organ."[64]

The Problems with Eating Meat

You may now understand why the great philosophers and spiritual geniuses of antiquity practiced fasting – and often for 40 days or more. They realized that darkness in their own consciousness inhibited their potential exalted states of consciousness, and that darkness was anchored to the filth in their own bodies. The dark thoughts of hate, anger, fear, etc. profoundly inhibit love, joy, peace, and enlightenment. As long as the dark unresolved issues remain within us, a heavy weight holds us low. Herein is the key **as to why the great spiritual genius would never indulge in the barbaric act of semi-cannibalistic consumption of innocent creatures of God, for the negative feelings of fear, hate, and death vibrate throughout the animal as it is being murdered.** Who would want to acquire and assimilate that?

There are clinical studies that support this concept.[65] Scientists found a way to train worms. After training worms to perform certain

---

[64] All of Dr. Anderson's books are available from Christobe Publishing, P.O. Box 1320, Mt. Shasta, CA. 96067. (530) 926-8855.

[65] Regarding the most outstanding experiment on rats, see Georges Unger, "Peptides and Memory," *Biochemistry Pharmacology,* 1974; May; Vol. 23, Number 11, pg. 1553-1558.
Regarding worms, see James J. McConnell, "Memory Transfer Through Cannibalism in Planaria," *Journal of Neuropsychiatry,* 1962; Volume 3, Supplement 1, pg. S42-48. The Medical establishment was shocked at this research and authorities subsequently did everything in their power to discredit all experimentation along these lines. But recent studies now support the validity of ideas explored in these initial experiments. For current information on this topic, see *Molecules of Emotion: The Science Behind Mind-Body Medicine,* by Candace B. Pert, Ph.D. (New York, NY: Touchstone, 1999).

behaviors that untrained worms were unable to exhibit, they ground up the trained worms and fed them to the untrained worms. Within a short time, the untrained worms were able to perform the same function just as the trained worms had, but without being trained. They absorbed the consciousness of the first group of worms, via their meat. Then scientists experimented with rats in a similar way. After injecting a preparation from the brains of the trained rats into the untrained rats, untrained rats easily performed the same learned behaviors as the trained rats without being trained.

The significance of course is obvious: **Animals and humans acquire the consciousness of whatever is within that which they eat.** If we eat an animal, **we actually absorb a portion of the animal's consciousness and it integrates with our own** – its fear, anger, **resentment, and its limitations.** As you can see, the old saying that we are what we eat does have significance.

I love animals; in fact, I have such love and respect for animals that I will never order their death by purchasing pieces of their bodies and eating them. But I also know the fear and anger they possess, and also their limited capacity to think deeply and to love one another. Have you ever witnessed an animal viciously fight another of its own specie over food or territory? Can you see now why the world is so degraded, so low, so competitive, so war-like, so materialistic and competitive? We live in a world dominated by meat eaters. There also may be other factors, but certainly this is a contributing factor.

It took me one year after I quit eating meat, in 1971, and several fasts before I finally rid myself of an anxiety associated with subtle fear and anger, and the seeming inability to find peace within. If you're still a meat eater and think you are happy, give up meat-eating for a year and one-half; cleanse or fast a few times, and you will find a peace and happiness you never knew existed. Not only that, but many people will learn more about how to love, **for the willingness to murder the innocent creatures of God for the unnecessary gluttony of ingesting animal flesh, and for the selfish appeasement of habits and taste buds, is in direct opposition to a loving and compassionate heart.**

How can we ever expect healing or continued health when **we willingly choose to steal the life and health of another creature for our own selfish gain?** Is there a law of cause and effect? Do we reap that which we sow?[66] Is there a law of Karma? Is it true that for every action

---

[66] Jesus said: ". . . and as they have sown in one life, so shall they reap in another." *The Gospel of the Perfect Life,* 94:4.

there is a reaction? If we are subject to these universal laws, then with a little reflection it becomes obvious that love is the greatest healing power and the wisest and most intelligent energy that we could ever use. For we know, even from a medical viewpoint, that love heals, strengthens, and energizes. **It is only through enough love that the Universe can flow through us, and truly heal us.** The great Master said, "Love thine enemies as thyself." Most people can't even love their own self. However, when we truly know what the self is, we will include all life, even animals, for we are life, not a body or even a mind. Love is giving, not stealing. Love is compassionate and assisting, not murderous; and love is for all life, not just for humans.[67]

Do Not Eat While Upset

Just as one can assimilate the fear from an animal by ingesting it, **we also assimilate the emotions *we* are feeling as we eat food**, and it appears that proteins are the magic glue that bind the emotions to our bodies. It's like producing a recording on a tape or hard drive, except that it continues to play, unconsciously, over and over until we remove it. Is it any wonder that habits and "ruts" are so difficult to change? Truly, we should never eat when we are dealing with stressful feelings. Refuse to do so from this moment forward!

---

[67] Jesus said: "Behold, I manifest myself unto you, in all created forms; and verily I say unto you, Inasmuch as ye have done it unto the least of these my brethren, ye have done it unto me." *The Gospel of the Perfect Life,* 67:10. He also said, in verse 19:6, **"Raise the Stone, and there thou shall find me. Cleave the wood, and there am I. For in the fire and in the water even as in every living form, God is manifest as its Life and its Substance."** A similar quote is also found in the *Gospel of Thomas* translated by Marvin W. Meyer: **"Split a piece of wood, and I am there. Pick up a stone, and you will find me there."** The *Gospel of Thomas* was only 1 of 52 texts known as the Nag Hammadi manuscripts found in upper Egypt in December 1945. Source: *The Secret Teachings Of Jesus: Four Gnostic Gospels,* translated by Marvin W. Meyer, (New York: Random House, 1984).

The Gospel of the Perfect Life reports that Jesus also said, **"I am come to end the sacrifices and feasts of blood, and if ye cease not offering and eating of flesh and blood, the wrath of God shall not cease from you, even as it came to your fathers in the wilderness, who lusted for flesh, and they eat to their content, and were filled with rottenness, and the plaque consumed them."** *The Gospel of the Perfect Life,* 21:8.

71

CHAPTER 5

PARASITES: ATTRACTED BY FILTHY BODIES

"How can a truly clean person possibly become infested with parasites? He can't."

– Rich Anderson, N.D., N.M.D.

There are approximately 130 species of parasites that can live in the human body. Many people believe that a large percentage of Americans host one kind or another. One medical parasitology textbook reported in 1989 that **over 55 million American children are infected with worms and that this is a gross underestimation if one includes parasites such as** pinworms, **for pinworms are the most common parasite among American children.** Now, that amazed even me, for that number implies that most children are infected. This textbook also reported that a doctor in Amherst, Massachusetts claimed that over the years of his practice he had treated virtually every major parasitic dis-ease of humans.[68]

Parasites can be the cause of serious malnutrition. Children suffering malnutrition and intestinal infection, caused by parasites, amount to 25% of worldwide deaths. Parasite epidemics have occurred in New York, Colorado, Washington, and New Hampshire, with serious outbreaks in other states. **Some common worms such as** roundworms **lay over 200,000 eggs a day.** Hookworms **lay 5,000 to 10,000 eggs a day and can live for about fourteen years.** They are prolific breeders.

Each parasite has its own unique action. *E. histolytica* destroys the intestinal wall by extruding proteolytic enzymes. *Fasciolopsis buski* causes damage to the intestinal wall by its powerful suckers. *Ascaris lumbricodes* can also perforate the gut wall, and invade the appendix, bile duct, and other organs. It can also cause severe constipation by blocking or plugging the alimentary canal. Hookworms suck blood and drain iron reserves, causing anemia. Tapeworms and other parasites compete nutritionally, draining the host of essential B vitamins, especially B-12, and other essential elements. Some parasites can coat the inside lining of the small

---

[68] Gerald K. Schmidt and Larry S. Roberts, *Foundations of Parasitology*, (St. Louis, MO: Times Mirror/Mosby College Publishing, 1989).

intestine and prevent the lining from absorbing nutrients in food. On a worldwide basis, worms outrank cancer as man's deadliest enemy. In fact, the World Health Organization has named parasitic dis-eases among the six most harmful infective dis-eases in humans.

In 1991 it was estimated that 1.2 billion people were infected with *Ascaris lumbricodes*. Ascaris is one of the largest worms that affects humans – up to two feet long. The largest, however, are tapeworms – over 30 feet long. Children and dogs are most affected.

In Brazil one parasite, *American Trypanosomiasis*, causes 30% of adult deaths. Relative to other countries, it was thought that North Americans suffered little from parasitic dis-eases because of our "good health," "good nutrition," climate, and sanitation. Climate, yes, sanitation, yes, but the fact that we are one of the sickest nations in the world reflects poor nutrition. Increasingly poor eating habits are plaguing each new generation, and along with this comes an increase of parasites. Parasitic dis-eases in America have increased significantly just in the last two decades – and will probably increase exponentially in the next two generations. Few medical doctors understand the significance of this. Seldom do they look for parasites in their patients. And even if they suspect parasites, few can effectively identify and treat them.

I knew a doctor who was examining a patient's eyes with an optical microscope and saw a tiny worm crawl from one part of the eye to the other side and disappear. Parasites may be microscopic in size or as long as 30 feet (or longer). Only a few are deadly, but they can cause a great deal of trouble. **Symptoms of parasite infestation mimic many other dis-eases, thereby avoiding accurate diagnosis**.

Parasites can live anywhere in the body – the lungs, liver, lymph glands, heart, prostate, bile ducts, skin, appendix, muscles, brain – but most abide in the intestinal tract. One autopsy of one woman revealed five tapeworms in her head. If they cause damage to the nerves in the head or spine, symptoms can occur anywhere in the body, from one end to the other. Similarly, if worms are in the intestinal tract, they can cause problems in the heart, liver, kidneys, brain, etc. by their toxic secretions or by reflex disturbance.

Most doctors never test for parasites, and most of the ones who do, fail to do it correctly. Apparently they fail to take parasites seriously, even though their own journals and textbooks reveal that they should. The stool test, their standard procedure, has proven only 39% effective. Experts test a mucoid plaque smear, which has proven most effective for discovering intestinal parasites.

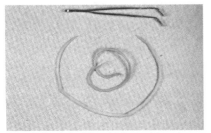

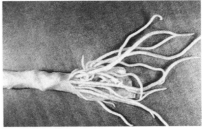

Ascaris lumbricoides: Male and female adults. Large, pinkish-white. Female is 22 to 35 centimeters long; male is 10 to 31 centimeters long. Females lay up to 250,000 eggs per day. Life span, more than 1 year. Adult worms may be passed in feces. Severe infection can cause pneumonia or death. Know as the "large intestinal roundworm."

Section of Bowel Obstructed with Ascaris lumbricoides: This parasite is found worldwide, though is more common in tropical climates.

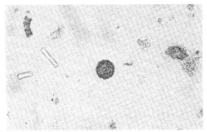

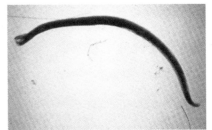

Ascaris lumbricoides Egg: Some species may be carried by dogs and cats, and are often passed to children via contact with infected soil. Cause inflammatory reactions leading to occlusions of capillaries in vital organs such as eyes, liver, brain, lungs. Magnified 100x.

Adult Male Hookworm: Magnified 10x. Small, grayish-white nematode (a roundworm). Females approximately 12 millimeters long, males approximately 9 millimeters. Females produces 5,000 to 10,000 eggs per day, and can live up to 14 years!

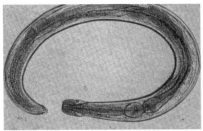

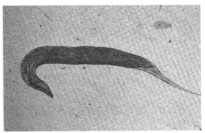

Male Pinworm: Magnified 20x. 2 to 5 millimeters long. Female migrates from colon to perianal area to deposit her eggs. Causes severe rectal itching.

Female Pinworm: Magnified 10x. 8 to 13 millimeters long. Female migrates from colon to perianal area to deposit her eggs. Causes severe rectal itching.

Following is a partial list of parasite dis-ease symptoms. Do you ever have symptoms like these?

Abdominal pain	Jaundice
Acute muscular inflammation	Joint pain
Acute, chronic constipation	Loss of sleep
Anemia	Lung and bronchial
Anorexia	congestion
B-12 deficiency	Malaria-like chills and
Bleeding rectum	fevers
Blindness	Malnutrition
Blood in feces	Muscle pain/spasms
Bloody spit	Nausea
Blurry vision	Night sweating
Burning urination	Pain in appendix area
Burping	Pain in guts
Central nervous system impairment	Poor memory
Chest pains	Mental problems,
Chills	Rashes
Chronic fatigue	Rectal prolapsus
Colitis	Short of breath
Coughing	Skin ulcers
Diarrhea	Sweating
Digestive disturbance	Swelling of eyes, face, etc.
Disfigurement of various body parts	Typhoid fever symptoms
Dizziness	Vomiting
Fevers	Weak immunity
Headaches	Weakness
Irritability	Weight gain
Itching	Weight loss
Enlargement and malfunction of organs such as liver, spleen, lymph nodes, heart, gallbladder, etc. Vaginal inflammation with yellow, frothy, foul-smelling discharges[69]	

You may be asking how a clean-living person could possibly become infested with parasites. Taking a shower does not mean that one is clean on the inside. What does your breath smell like in the morning? If your mouth is sweet and pleasurably kissable, then maybe you're clean. If it is otherwise, you've created a condition that can or has attracted parasites. Junk and processed foods, and foods fried in oils, including French fries, are like magnets to parasites, for these so-called "foods" overwork and weaken the stomach, pancreas, kidneys, liver, heart, and other organs. They

---

[69] For a list of symptoms associated with conventional medical treatments for parasites read *Cleanse & Purify Thyself*, Book 2.

severely strain the body's immune system, help create mucoid plaque and produce the ideal breeding ground for parasites. Meat and fish are major sources of parasites. Parasite eggs are extremely resistant to heat and cold. Unless meat is extremely overcooked, the eggs survive. Some of the more serious infections (especially those involving large worms) find their way into the human body when one eats cooked pork, beef, fish, or any other creatures that have eyeballs, legs, fins, or pinchers (yes, that includes crab and lobster). And if you eat these sea "insects," not only does your breath smell bad in the morning, but also you probably feel the need to use deodorants, perfumes, and colognes. Touching infected dogs, cats, and other animals may also lead to one's picking up parasite eggs or even parasites themselves. Other methods of infection are listed below.[70]

♦ Drinking or swimming in infected water
♦ Being bitten by flies, mosquitoes, ticks, or animals
♦ Contacting filthy environments through breathing or touching (remember, just like cockroaches, parasites thrive in a filthy environment)
♦ Eating foods grown in infected soil, especially soil which has been fertilized with pig dung
♦ Eating water chestnuts
♦ Walking barefooted on infected soil

Parasites and worms thrive in mucoid layers and filth. They feed on it, they are protected by it, and they contribute to the toxicity of mucoid plaque and the body as a whole. Vermifuges (de-worming products) have great difficulty penetrating the mucin barrier. Parasites thrive beneath the mucoid plaque, happily nestled in their perfect habitat. Until the plaque is removed once and for all, bowel pH returned to normal, the correct bacteria rule the intestinal environment, the diet is cleaned up, our digestive system functions normally, and the intestinal immune function kicks back in, worms and parasites have a good chance for a long life. **For parasites thrive upon undigested proteins and processed foods that contribute towards a filthy internal environment.**

Once parasites are in the body, the only sure way to get them out is to get rid of the environment of filth that they feed upon. Have you ever seen flies in a clean garbage can? Take away their food and they will go away, especially with the help of herbal vermifuges and with strengthening the liver and the immune system. Remember the promise and take heart: "Cleanse and purify thyself and I will exalt thee to the throne of power!" And long before you recognize *that* throne of power, you will recognize the *porcelain* throne of power.

---

[70] As noted on page 20, the "diamond bullets" indicate warning points.

Years ago I suspected that I might have a tapeworm – and who knew what else. I tried various remedies with no obvious results. Later, Dr. Jensen explained that the only truly effective means he knew of to eliminate worms was to eat nothing but raw onions and garlic for three days and then to take a strong herbal laxative (overdose) on the last night. His directions included sitting in warm milk the next morning, when it was time for bowel movement. Worms love milk. The theory is that the weakened worms will end up in the colon after fleeing from the raw onion and garlic, but scurry back up when feeling the cold air at the anus. If they sense the warm milk instead, they will go for it.

I often explored the effectiveness of various remedies and herbs with my expert herbalist friend, White Crow. And, since I never recommended anything that I hadn't tried myself, I convinced Crow to take off for the mountains with me, to try this remedy. We went through three days of agony and even sat in the warm milk. The last part was the most hilarious moment of my life but that shall remain unwritten. The only thing that came out was a one-inch hookworm. I have never recommended this procedure to anyone.

About a year later I was in Tucson, cleansing and experimenting with eating one meal a day. I had made tremendous progress in cleansing, but I still had a long way to go and much to learn. The only part of my digestive system that was not completely free of mucoid plaque was the stomach, and perhaps a few other small areas here and there (where I held stuck emotions). I was certain of this because I still had an apparent hydrochloric acid deficiency and there was one little spot of discoloration on my tongue that hadn't yet cleared.[71] It was the fourth day of my cleanse and I had just finished taking a psyllium and bentonite shake when unexpectedly I suddenly gulped for air. I doubled over and grabbed my stomach. For about 20 minutes I held my stomach and was unable to stand up straight. It felt like something was trying to turn my stomach inside out. It wasn't painful, but it was a very weird feeling. Then, just as suddenly as it had come, it disappeared and never returned. The next morning I passed a worm that was about four feet long. The morning after that, I passed either another worm, or a piece of the previous one that was about a foot long. So, once you start cleansing seriously, be aware that such an experience may happen to you. And be thankful if it does.

---

[71] Chinese medicine uses tongue analysis to help reveal conditions in other parts of the body. Similar to the iris, but not nearly as complex, the tongue reflects conditions in the stomach, liver, and other areas of our body.

One woman who had to deal with parasites swore that our Cleanse and anti-parasite program were responsible for saving her life. Within a week after she began her cleanse, worms began to evacuate her body by the cupfuls. She would call and tell my staff what was happening, and it was almost unbelievable. *At night, worms even came out through her mouth and nose.* Cups of worms came out every day until she finished the Cleanse. In a few weeks she did another cleanse and this time used my de-worming program. And once again worms flooded her toilet. For about a year and a half worms continued to leave her body, and she became stronger and stronger. Finally, the worms stopped appearing, and she had achieved a state of health that exceeded her expectations. A few years later I met her and her husband. With tears and hugs, they expressed their deepest appreciation for me, and our Cleanse. She said that the Cleanse had been her last hope, for no doctor or treatment had been able to help her.

Why Focus on Intestinal Cleansing – What About Other Kinds of Cleansing?

As the bowel controls the assimilation process, it also has a great influence upon the body's elimination process. Remember, **the bowel is the hub** of our body. The bowel may be likened to a septic system in a house. If your leach line becomes clogged, you may find septic debris flooding into your bathtub or shower, especially after that one last flush. In a similar way, when the bowel is congested, the blood and lymph also become backed up, similarly to how it happens with a septic system. For, more bulk waste is removed from the bowel than from any other elimination organ. When it becomes clogged, it will be felt in every cell and organ and especially noticed in the blood and lymph. When the circulatory systems are unable to release their waste efficiently, they are also unable to keep up with the toxic waste from cellular metabolism, – unable to carry the toxic waste to the needed exit point, so that even the cells become backed up and congested.

With the use of a powerful medical microscope we can easily examine the blood before and after cleansing, and the difference is obvious at a glance. Not only is there less debris, but the action of the white blood cells is truly amazing. Prior to cleansing, the white blood cells in most people move about like slugs in a garden or turtles slowly crawling through an obstacle course. **After cleansing, the white blood cells move more freely, approximately 4 to 10 times the velocity prior to cleansing.** The sluggishness prior to cleansing appears to be the result of excessive mucus and proteins in the blood, which the body should have removed, but couldn't. When the bowel is free of congestion, the internal fluids, primarily the lymph and blood, are much more capable of picking up toxic waste and carrying it to one of the elimination organs (bowel, skin, kidneys, and lungs) and then removing it once and forever. Many times I have observed that white blood cells (immune cells) that are distorted before cleansing become normal after cleansing.

Cancer cannot live in a body with a strong immune system, nor can parasites. When we have a strong immune system, we have a strong body; everything is in working order. That means a strong digestive system, maximum hydrochloric acid, alkaline bile, and alkaline blood. As Dr. Jensen used to say, "If you step on a cat's tail, it's the other end that yells." He implies with this that the whole body is connected and works synergistically with every other part. This is wisdom seldom found in conventional medicine. For the effective treatment for any dis-ease, one should treat the whole body, not just an isolated part or aspect of it.

I have used almost every cleansing program available, including blood, bowel, and liver cleansers, as well as numerous kidney, brain, and gallbladder cleanses. I also accomplished skin and lymph cleansing. I have used hundreds of different herbs, homeopathics, sweats, foods, juices, water, exercises, electronic equipment, etc. **And nothing, absolutely nothing, works the magic of a superb intestinal cleanse.** Not only that, but **all other programs work much more effectively after one has accomplished serious intestinal cleansing.**

CHAPTER 6

HOW I DEVELOPED MY CLEANSING PROGRAM

"For know that true knowledge is alone to be found in your own soul, and the way to your soul is through the passage of the heart, from which all darkness must be banished by the light of selflessness."

– Rich Anderson, N.D., N.M.D.

I started colon cleansing with a very well known program that claimed "no cleansing reactions." After a month of feeling more sluggish and rather depressed and without experiencing a single positive result, I dropped it like a hot potato. I began researching and using other herbal colon cleansing programs and finally obtained what I then thought were great results – an average of 13 feet of mucoid plaque came out of me in seven days, and I can assure you that wasn't just your average fecal excretions! Then Dr. Bernard Jensen convinced me to try pancreatin, which resulted in the elimination of 28 feet in seven days. However, pancreatin is an animal product, and I was determined to find something as or more effective without putting the death vibration of a slaughtered animal into my body. With that intent, I sent a little prayer to help me find something pure that would allow me to achieve complete purification of my alimentary canal, which then would help facilitate the purification of my whole being.

The next summer, I scheduled a research and experimentation expedition with my old friend – White Medicine Crow. We planned to live off the land, eating only wild, fresh herbs; live in the open air; sleep under the stars (no tent); take cold baths in streams and lakes; and study the human soul. We started in the Arizona mountainous desert and almost starved to death - not because we couldn't find food, but because the food tasted terrible. After becoming sick from bad water, we went to the Sierra Nevada Mountains in California, which was heavenly. Then we proceeded to the Redwoods, the ocean, and finally the North Cascades in Washington.

We were still very ill after we arrived in the Sierras; in fact, we could hardly walk. Our only food, besides fresh wild herbs, was apple cider vinegar, a few lemons, and raisins to help dress up our herbal salads. We ate two meals daily. We would take our empty wooden bowls and walk out into a meadow or woods and carefully pick a variety of herbs until our bowls were full. Then we'd take them back to camp, add dressing, and then gobble down our health-giving herbs.

We had been eating herbs from one particular meadow for about four or five days when the following experience took place: I was sitting upon a rock reading a book near our teepee, which was made from cedar bark. White Crow had gone for a walk and was out of sight. Suddenly, I heard him yelling. "Rich, come quick. Rich, come up here, run!"

I thought, "What's happening? Was he bitten by a rattlesnake?" I dropped my book and ran as fast as I could in his direction (which wasn't all that fast, considering my miserable condition).

When I reached him he pointed to the earth and said, "Look!"

There lying on the ground was a long narrow blackish grey snake-like mass about four feet long. At first I thought that he had killed a rattlesnake and wondered immediately if he had been bitten. Then calmly he said, "Is this one of those mucoid layers you've been telling me about?"

I quickly evaluated the situation; it was not a snake. Looking a little more carefully, I saw that it looked like a piece of long leather or rubber-like rope. After my examination I fully realized that it was indeed mucoid plaque, for its appearance clearly displayed the exact configurations of the intestinal wall. But, another mystery struck me. This hunk of mucoid plaque hadn't come from the colon; **it had come from the small intestines**. In fact, judging by its shape, structure, and striations, I knew it was from the upper intestines - from the jejunum, to be exact, which is just below the duodenum.

"What is going on here?" I thought. I had read every book on the subject that I could lay my hands on, and none had ever discussed plaque coming from the small intestines, only from the colon. Crow saw my bafflement.

"Well, what is it? Is it part of my guts, or what?" he persisted.

I thought quickly, for this was most unusual. Finally, I replied, "Yes indeed, that's mucoid plaque. Congratulations. You are now cleaner and healthier because that is on the outside instead of your inside. You will feel better, be stronger, and think more clearly. "But," I said in confusion, "you're not on a cleanse, so why in the world did this come out of you?" Before the day was over, he had released more plaque and so had I.

81

Soon, with every bowel movement, we both found rubber-like ropes, usually about two to four feet long, with the exact configurations of the intestinal wall. They were coming from all parts of the alimentary canal - the duodenum, jejunum, ileum, and the colon (except the stomach; that came later). I began to take this very seriously. By the second day of this massive cleansing we were pleased to find that our health and strength had returned. I contemplated this experience carefully. Here we were - consuming two large meals a day of fresh wild herbs. There was nothing else that could work this magic. It had become obvious that we had come upon a group of herbs that had tremendous healing potential. More and more I realized that this could be a very important discovery for anyone who had the wisdom to partake of it.

During the next ten days, our convalescence was rapid and so was the elimination of this dis-ease-causing plaque. We wondered if it would ever end. Our health, just in those ten days, had improved beyond our greatest expectations. Neither of us had ever felt better. Our energy increased daily; we steadily felt better and better. My eyesight improved, along with my mental abilities. Our meditation had become more profound. And along with everything else, our happiness also increased.

I persistently studied the herbs to determine which of them were responsible for this incredible cleansing. Most of the herbs we had been eating were common and well-known herbs. However, we were unaware of any herb that would release mucoid plaque to this proportion, or of any medical text that discussed anything about such an herb. Were we the first people in history to discover such a radical and profound cleansing activity? What was the potential here? If I could determine how to initiate this cleansing process, and control it, could it be a key to "cure" the incurables?

The next step, I thought, was to discover whether or not I could produce the same results using dried herbs instead of fresh ones. After all, hundreds of herbalists knew about the herbs we were ingesting, but apparently none of them had obtained these results. Why? Of course very few, if any, had gone into the wilderness and eaten only fresh wild herbs. It is possible, I thought, that the reason for this impressive cleansing is that the herbs are in their fresh raw state, with all the chlorophyll, vitality, life force, liquids, and enzymes at full strength. But something inside told me that it would work in the dried state just as well as in the fresh. If only I could figure out the right combination and the right amounts, and duplicate this powerful cleansing, I could perform a mighty service to mankind. I became almost possessed with the desire to learn more. I then planned to work on a formula that would help all who desired greater health.

By the time we finished our research in the North Cascades, I knew the combination of herbs, and there were several that were needed to produce the desired effect. After we had returned to Mt. Shasta, and our three-month expedition of eating off the land was completed, we settled down and I began to experiment with the formulation of dried herbs. Finding the correct proportions was a challenge. To put it mildly, we went through many uncomfortable cleansing reactions. One time we found that our brains were detoxifying at an extreme rate, and we could barely walk or function. One time we were camped on an ocean beach and Crow saw an otter walk out of the ocean, heading straight for us, which is an incredible event that I would never want to miss. He whispered for me to look, but I could barely raise my head to see him – the results of too much of one particular herb. After several adjustments I finally created the formula that would activate the cleansing and avoid unpleasant sensations. Now all I had to do was test it.

I developed a six-day program, which Crow volunteered to follow along with me. Everything went perfectly until the fourth day: In the middle of the night, White Crow arose and went to the kitchen and cooked up a large batch of potatoes. He had a pleasant feast, but it slowed down his Cleanse. However, he still was able to rid himself of 28 feet of the terrible mucoid plaque. He was so pleased with his results that he went around telling people how much plaque he had removed, and how wonderful he felt. Abstaining from the potatoes, I was able to eliminate 40 feet.

I'll never forget the day we stopped at an herb shop in Seattle. White Crow struck up a conversation with the owner, who was very proud of a colon cleanse that he had developed. This fellow was totally convinced that his cleanse was the best in the country. White Crow began describing the results we had with our recent cleanse experiment, and mentioned passing 28 feet of mucoid plaque in 6 days. I'll never forget that fellow's face! I walked over and told him about my 40 feet. His jaw dropped open. Then he turned and walked away without a word.

My wife's first cleanse was just as successful. Having only done one other "cleanse" before and passing no mucoid plaque at all, she was only doing my new cleanse to appease me. In seven days she passed 37 feet of the old, mucoid gunk and a few parasites. She was so thrilled she continued to cleanse about every seven weeks and intends to keep cleansing until nothing more comes out! It was amazing, also, how soft and smooth her skin became.

White Crow, my wife and I spent 45 days camped upon Mt. Shasta and one day I was inspired to write this book. It took 13 days. I have revised it several times, but it is still basically the same book. After the first edition in 1987, sales exploded. People would reluctantly follow my Cleanse, but after experiencing the unexpected results, they would give my book to their friends and relatives. Some people would purchase dozens of books and give them to their friends and students and associates. Soon, without any advertising, the book was purchased by people in more than 56 foreign countries. It wasn't because the book was so spectacular; it was because the program really works.

In those days we never used bentonite or psyllium: The psyllium-bentonite shakes were added a year or so later, to help minimize cleansing reactions in people who were highly toxic. Over the years I was able to fine-tune our program – truly a story in itself. Now after more than a decade, tens of thousands of people have used this program with spectacular results.

A few years later, many people and many companies began developing and selling their own cleansing programs. Many were attempting to duplicate our program, but no other program has equaled the results of my two special formulas, which evolved out of the experience I had in the Sierra Nevada Mountains, which I have just recounted.

We were informed by friends in Germany that one man from San Jose, California, was selling his cleanse in Europe and telling people that he was a personal friend of mine and that I had helped him formulate his products. I had never even heard the fellow's name before. My two biggest concerns, however, were not related to competition. I was pleased that I had been an instrument in bringing the awareness of cleansing to so many people. But I was concerned that many of the programs were frauds. People were selling products that simply did not work, and it made cleansing – and alternative medicine – look bad.

But my worst concern was what the pharmaceutical companies, and their principal American defender, the FDA (enemy of natural products and alternative medicine, and guardian of drugs) might do if they were to discover just how successful our program really was.[72] Unfortunately, we

---

[72] Approximately 400,000 Americans are killed and over 2 million are rushed to the emergency room each year because of medical drugs, and the FDA does nothing to curtail their use. But when a couple of people become ill because of an herb or other natural supplements, the FDA announces to the world how dangerous the product is. Without thorough and unbiased investigation, FDA officials do all in their power to eliminate any product that could compete with drugs, even when there is evidence that the natural product was not at fault. Examples include comfrey, lobelia, chapparrel, tryptophane, and various homeopathics.

learned that large numbers of people were told the lie that one of my primary formulas was dangerous; the FDA failed to notify the public what their own labs verified, that the problem was one of mysterious contamination, not formulation! In addition, the FDA curiously failed to report both that the contamination was confined to certain very limited batches, and also that the problem was quickly remedied and all customers immediately notified. Even in the year 2000, people have found that inaccurate notices remain on the Internet – results of the FDA's campaign – that propagated and perpetuated the lie. And of course many unscrupulous competitors took advantage of this and made derogatory remarks against both my product and myself, solely to increase their own profits.

It turns out that one herb in my formula, plantain, had mysteriously been contaminated with *digitalis lanata* in certain isolated batches. This is an herb (foxglove) used by pharmaceutical companies to produce the drug Digitalis, which is used to treat heart disease. Thousands of people believed the lies, and many believed that I was a scoundrel who deliberately deceived and poisoned the users of my products. Nothing, absolutely nothing, could be further from the truth. Though we long ago had known about the corruption of the FDA and its intimate relationship with drug companies, we unfortunately had to experience its power and the power of the press to attempt to destroy a wonderful thing. But this is another story.

Formula 1

The keys to the success of my Cleansing Program are two herbal formulas. The first one I nicknamed the *"Intestinal Reamer Cleaner."* It was designed to achieve the following results[73]:

❑ Dissolve and break up mucoid plaque
❑ Rapidly expel mucoid plaque from the system
❑ Cause no cramping
❑ Reduce gas in the stomach and intestines
❑ Kill any possible infection and heal any sore areas
❑ Purify the blood to help reduce cleansing reactions
❑ Help strengthen, heal and re-build peristalsis
❑ Reduce appetite
❑ Remove some worms
❑ Stop any hemorrhages in case polyps or tumors are torn away from the gut wall.

---

[73] As noted on page 20, the "box bullets" indicate informational points.

Formula 2

This formula contains several of the herbs that help produce the "magic." With this formula, I added several important herbs to help protect and support the body while cleansing. This formula is full of nutritional herbal power. It was designed to supply the following:

- ❑ Vitamins and minerals in their natural combinations
- ❑ Essential amino acids
- ❑ Vitamin C, calcium, iron, and potassium
- ❑ Stimulation of and support to the lymph system
- ❑ Vitamins A and B
- ❑ Chlorophyll
- ❑ Support and strength for all organs, especially the heart, liver, and eliminative organs

When this nutritional herbal formula eventually came to the point where I was satisfied with all those requirements, I knew it was a fantastic product. Every vitamin and mineral supplement I knew of on the market seemed seriously out of balance with Nature. It therefore seemed clear that anyone who knew much about Nature, vitamins, minerals, buffering agents, drugs, the dissection of natural ingredients, combinations, digestion, assimilation, and the meaning of organic versus inorganic would be much happier with this formula than with what was generally found on the market.

What to Expect While Cleansing

When using our program, the average piece of mucoid plaque expelled is 6 to 18 inches long, and it is not uncommon to expel pieces more than two to four (2-4) feet long. Some people report the elimination of worms. During the first two cleanses it is common to see yellowish-white popcorn-like pieces or flakes (polyps), or an amber or dark green, jelly-like goop (lymph). Fun stuff! This is where cleansing becomes entertaining and educational. You will soon consider yourself a qualified "intestinal discharge examiner."

For years I kept a pair of chopsticks by my "porcelain throne," for they assisted my examination and ease in measuring the mucoid plaque. If several family members or friends cleanse at the same time, it's fun to keep track of the number of feet removed and compare notes. No kidding! It's at least ten times more entertaining than the average TV sitcom and enormously more valuable. Looking into the toilet and scrutinizing that dis-ease-potential substance, you will be filled with great joy, for you will be flushing away one of the primary causes of lack of energy, premature old age, failing eyesight, poor memory, and dis-ease elements. Discharges may flow from any and all channels of elimination during the Cleanse – the kidneys, skin, lungs, mouth, nose, and ears. The average amount of plaque removed during the first two or three cleanses is about 25 to 50 feet. It is no wonder that after cleansing, people experience more energy and new attitudes, and no wonder that the number-two testimony we have heard over the years has been, "After completing your Cleanse I feel closer to God and much more loving."

More than One Cleanse?

The plaque and other foul matter that can be removed during a seven-day period (during the Master Phase) are astonishing to most people. And you should enjoy a noticeable improvement in your health within a few days after cleansing. However, for most people one four-week cleanse, including one week of the Master Phase, will not remove all the mucoid plaque from the intestinal tract. Many, many years have been spent building layer upon layer of this substance throughout the entire alimentary canal. There is no telling how thick the layers have become. On a thin person, the layers may be one-fourth of an inch thick; a heavy person tends to accumulate more. One colon was known to be 18 inches thick in diameter! Less than 5% of cleansers report no mucoid plaque removed, and most of these people report other benefits. Six to eight weeks after your first cleanse, another cleanse may be started.

Note: If you are following the milder phases, you can cleanse much more often.

As a rule, I recommend that three or four cleanses be accomplished during the first year, and two per year thereafter. Many people have cleansed much more than that, with excellent results. I have found in myself, and from observing others that our bodies yearn to be cleansed in the way I recommend, but after the mucoid plaque is gone, the body stops encouraging it and we automatically lose the desire to cleanse in this manner.

If this program is followed and nutritious eating habits are maintained, a state of health can be achieved that may amaze you. This has been found to be true of people even 80 years and older. This depends on the factors listed below:

- ❑ Your current condition,
- ❑ How closely you follow the Cleanse instructions,
- ❑ How well you eat between cleanses, and
- ❑ Which phase you follow.

Right now you may be thinking, "I'm not even sure I want to do one cleanse, let alone several a year." To you, my friend, let me simply encourage you to try it for the first time. Even if you do the Cleanse only once a year, you will be giving your body enormous relief, saving it from the tiresome task of spending all its energy digesting and protecting itself from the overload of toxic matter we thoughtlessly dump into it three times a day (this doesn't even include snacking and coffee breaks). How much is your health worth to you? This once-a-year vacation would give the body a chance to take a breather and devote its energy to healing itself. And, besides, you may change your mind once you complete the first cleanse. The most important thing is to muster your courage and venture a first step into the unknown. It's true, not everyone has the strength to do this. You will be distinguishing yourself from the lot of mankind who accept ill health as a cruel twist of fate, and unconsciously struggle through life, blindly accepting unnecessary suffering. You will be proud of yourself and will realize the "stuff" of which you are really made, once you have completed your first cleanse.

CHAPTER 7

BENEFITS OF COMPLETE INTESTINAL CLEANSING

"Perfect health is not only essential to this highest state of Bliss, but it is also an attribute of God."

– Dr. Rich Anderson

Cleansing the Entire Gastrointestinal Tract

An effective intestinal cleansing program will cleanse the entire gastrointestinal tract all the way from the tip of the tongue to the anus. The colon tends to accumulate a greater abundance of mucoid plaque than does the small intestine, but the small intestine is five times longer than the colon, and so the majority of what people see being eliminated will be from the small intestine.

Sections of the Intestines

The inner wall of the small intestines has extensive folds called plicae circularis. **These folds give the mucoid plaque the unique shapes and markings you see when pieces of mucoid plaque are expelled.** Their function is to churn the food so that all foodstuffs have the opportunity to touch the "brush border," and mix with the enzymes that are secreted through the epithelium wall. These folds expand the surface area by three times. Each fold contains numerous microscopic structures called villi, which expand the surface area another 10 times. Each villus consists of a single layer of surface epithelial cells and covers an inner core of tiny blood and lymph vessels, nerve fibers, and smooth muscle cells. In a healthy individual, each epithelial cell of the villus projects approximately 1000 microvilli. These microvilli, expand the surface another 20 times. Altogether, the plicae circularis, the villi, and the microvilli increase the absorptive surface **six hundred-fold, providing an area the size of a tennis court for nutrient absorption.**

But how many bowels are capable of allowing the "food stuff" to make contact with the "brush border," to absorb the needed digestive enzymes, and then to pass through the epithelium wall and into the blood? Mucoid plaque covering the epithelium wall also covers the folds, villi, and the microvilli. Obviously any layers of plaque could interfere with food reaching the intestinal wall. Oh, what "civilization," so-called, has done unto us.

The bottom layer of plaque takes on the exact shape of the intestinal wall, and the next layer takes on its shape. Observing the markings of mucoid plaque allows us to identify where it came from. For example, if the plaque came from the duodenum, you know that the secretions from the pancreas, liver, and gallbladder ducts (the source of many digestive enzymes) may have been blocked. Therefore, you can assume that your body's ability to digest fats and other foods may have been inhibited, but may now have been corrected.

Hopefully, your first cleanse will eliminate all obstructions in this area. If not on the first cleanse, maybe the next. But you see how important this could be. For if this area were covered with layers of mucoid fecal substance, the secretions from the digestive glands would flow underneath the mucoid matter, which would severely limit its contact with the food. Perhaps only a trickle of digestive fluids would actually contact your food. If the mucoid layers exerted sufficient pressure, a back-up could occur in the pancreatic and gallbladder ducts, as well as a back-up of all fluids that drain into the bowel. This could affect the liver and many other organs. Can you see how mucoid plaque may be related to gallbladder and pancreatic problems? And diabetes and hypoglycemia may also be related to bowel problems. The truth is, we don't know, but I put this forth as a speculative hypothesis, which may be proven true one day in the far future.

Most nourishment is assimilated in the small intestine, although some nourishment may be absorbed through the stomach and colon. If you were to notice mucoid substance coming from the jejunum and ileum, you would again know that your body's ability to assimilate food properly has been greatly impaired. You could have been eating the most perfect, organic foods to no avail. Along with the presence of the mucoid layers is usually an imbalanced intestinal flora. It is estimated that these toxic, undesirable microorganisms rule in the bowels of 85% of the American people. They produce sometimes-bizarre reactions and consistently break down healthy tissue and drain a person's energy. They are also the main cause of gas.

Some of these pathogenic bacteria are *Bacillus coli,* which have been known to cause cancer in laboratory animals. Most people who have cancer never find out why. It is interesting to note that cancer among meat eaters is about 90% *higher* than among lifelong vegetarians. And the primary sustenance of the *Bacillus coli* is meat. Next on the list of causes of cancer and ill health in general are acid-forming foods, overcooked foods and undigested proteins. Meat substitutes are high on the list of detrimental foods for vegetarians. Once the body is cleansed of the causes of the imbalance in intestinal flora, it becomes possible to replace harmful bacteria with "friendly bacteria." But even in this area, great mistakes are made. Acidophilus for many years has been thought to be the perfect bacteria for man. Undoubtedly, *Lactobacillus acidophilus* has an important part to play, for it can remove a variety of pathogens from the bowel. However, *Lactobacillus* **bacteria should be used only in treating a condition, not to replace the bacteria in our bowels**. *Acidophilus* is highly acid-forming; that is why its name includes the word "acid" in "*acidophilus*." This subject is thoroughly discussed in Chapter 9, under "Probiotics."

Absorption of Nutrients

The more mucoid plaque that is removed from our bowels, the better we can digest and absorb the nutrients from the food we eat. People are often surprised at how little food one really needs. Once "cleansed," a woman ate only one small meal every other day for two years. She reported that she had never felt so mentally alert and physically alive. Many toxic people absorb only a portion of the nutrients in their food – no matter how nutritious the food or how much they eat. Although a clean bowel is no guarantee that our digestion will be perfect, for there are many other factors involved, it certainly is a good start.

Increased Peristaltic Action of the Intestines

Many people experience increased peristalsis after cleansing, but not everyone. I have found that unresolved emotions affect peristalsis more than any other factor. Yet, it's obvious that mucoid plaque plays an important part in sluggish peristalsis and in constipation. When food moves through the bowels slowly, as in constipation, the fecal matter becomes firmer and dryer, and this is a precursor to fecal pockets, bulges, diverticulitis, and a host of other colon problems and dis-ease. Merck's Manual, the medical doctors' bible, states that over 98% of Americans will develop diverticulitis if they live long enough. I will not be in that statistical database, and I hope that you will avoid it also.

Removal of a Major Source of Dis-ease

A toxic bowel is the perfect breeding environment for billions of dis-ease related bacteria, germs, and parasites. This toxic bowel environment poisons the blood, the liver, and every cell of the body. Major organs are constantly being overloaded and working overtime, persistently compensating for the extreme stress placed upon the body. Intestinal cleansing removes pathogenic bacteria effectively and harmlessly. Antibiotics also remove pathogenic bacteria, but with a terrible cost to future health. Antibiotics, unfortunately, murder all the friendly and natural bacteria and will do nothing to alter the filthy environment that attracted the pathogens. Thorough cleansing changes our internal milieu. Removing mucoid plaque is also eliminating a major cause of putrefaction and fermentation. Intestinal cleansing allows a rapid repair of the damage done in the past. And the miracle of the body is that it will repair itself; all it requires is the freedom from congestion and toxins, and the proper nutrients. When no longer spent on constant adjustments, the energy in your body can be used for healing and for the mind. Marvelous ideas, clear thinking, joy, and love can predominate.

Improvement of Nerve Flow

It is well known that millions of nerves pass through the spinal column. When a vertebra is out of alignment, spinal nerves are pinched, which can seriously affect the organ or area that the nerve supplies. Similarly, but not so dramatically, there are nerve reflex points in the intestines. When the intestinal tract is gorged with fecal and mucoid impaction, nerves can short-circuit. This may be one reason why bowel impaction has such a tremendous influence upon organs that are seemingly unrelated to the bowel. The heart is a good example. The reflex points for the heart are in the descending colon. Dr. Jensen was the first to point this out to me. He explained that when he saw a dark spot in the area of the iris, he would ask his patient if he or she had any heart problems. Most of these people did. Then he asked them to massage deeply in the descending colon and find out if there were any sensitive areas. About 75% of the time they discovered there were sore spots. Later I used the same procedure and found that this 75% was consistent. If a person had a bowel pocket – mucoid plaque that has become impacted into the epithelium wall of the descending colon – that person was likely to have a heart condition. Removal of that bowel pocket usually resulted in a lessening of heart problems.

A splendid example is with hypertension (high blood pressure). Every person I have ever seen who had hypertension before cleansing found it became normal or had greatly improved after cleansing. I have won a few bets on this one.

Obliteration of Obesity

Among the main causes of obesity are trapped proteins, toxins and acids. When toxins and/or acids cannot escape faster than they are being produced, the body protects itself by wrapping the toxins with mucus or lymph, and stores them. The cleansing of the alimentary canal eliminates the pressure placed upon the lymphatic system, the blood, the brain, elimination organs, and the entire body. This allows the lymphatics and other organs to dump excesses. It is no wonder that cleansers enjoy greater health, energy, endurance, strength, and mental alertness.

I have on my desk a testimony of a man who weighed 308 pounds before starting my program and weighed 240 pounds after cleansing. He had severe constipation for 10 years, with bleeding, but now that condition has been overcome, and he is feeling wonderful!

Prolapsus Adjustment

Oftentimes, the weight and pressure of many layers of mucoid plaque, coupled with gravity over a period of time, may cause prolapsus of the transverse colon and the stomach. The stomach may drop into what is called a "fishhook" position and may cause further digestive problems by pooling stomach acids. Prolapsus of the transverse colon also exerts pressure on the lower organs and contributes towards bladder and urinary problems, various imbalances of the nerve centers, prostate ailments, and uterine and other female problems. All of these conditions may repair themselves after the removal of the mucoid plaque and with the use of certain herbs and exercises, as detailed in Chapter 10 under "How to Shrink the Abdomen, Repair Prolapsus."

Shrinking the Abdomen

As you can imagine, mucoid plaque can eventually stretch the intestinal wall, especially the colon. Those people displaying the famous "beer belly," or "Dunlap dis-ease", and others whose stomachs fold or have "done lapped" over the belt, or those who cannot see their feet when they stand up straight, can be sure that they have thick and dangerous mucoid build-up in the intestinal tract. This is generally a sign of a serious future dis-ease and shortened life span. This condition can be vastly improved or elimination by cleansing thoroughly.

See Chapter 10 in this book: "Important Facts about an Optimal Cleansing Program" for instructions on how to shrink the abdomen and help to repair a prolapsed colon.

The Iris of the Eye

Following is a chart on the science of how to read the markings in the iris of the eye – iridology. Each point of the iris reveals the condition of a corresponding part of the body. It reflects the various stages of cellular health: acute, subacute, chronic and degeneration. When people cleanse deeply, all the way to the cellular level, changes will reflect in the iris. It generally takes three or more weeks before changes in the body are reflected in the iris.

One lady I knew very well was born with brown eyes. She began using our program after her 44th year, and after five cleanses, the color of her eyes had become bluish green, with no trace of brown.

I have used both the sciences of iridology and hematology for many years; and as valuable as blood analysis has been to me, **I have found iris analysis to be even more useful;** and I have often used iridology to either substantiate or negate what I find in the blood. Iridology is very accurate if it is used properly. And what allows for proper use? Proper use requires a clear understanding that **every unnatural aspect found in the iris indicates two important facts: stuck emotions and toxicity**. It also requires knowing that these two conditions cause most of the problems in our bodies.

CHART ON IRIDOLOGY

IRIS-1
(Iridology)

©June 1996 by LEONARD MEHLMAUER, HP
Cammarillo, California, USA • 805-484-8686
e-mail: grandmedicine@vcnet.com

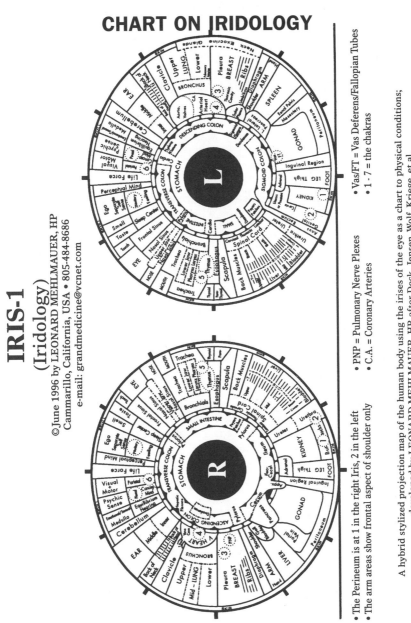

• The Perineum is at 1 in the right Iris, 2 in the left
• The arm areas show frontal aspect of shoulder only

• PNP = Pulmonary Nerve Plexes
• C.A. = Coronary Arteries

• Vas/FT = Vas Deferens/Fallopian Tubes
• 1 - 7 = the chakras

A hybrid stylized projection map of the human body using the irises of the eye as a chart to physical conditions;
developed by LEONARD MEHLMAUER, HP, after Deck, Jensen, Wolf, Kriege, et al.

CHAPTER 8

HOW TO DETERMINE IF YOU NEED THE CLEANSE

If you've been living on raw fruits and vegetables all your life, chances are you do not need the Cleanse. However, if you have any of the following, you are most likely in serious need of intestinal cleansing[74]:

♦ Any dis-ease or malfunction of the body.
♦ Constipation (less than 2 BM's daily).
♦ Bad breath.
♦ Body odor.
♦ Flatulence (gas).
♦ Dry and hard stools (they should be soft and break up when you flush).
♦ Foul-smelling stools (unless you eat onions or garlic) or off-color stools (they should be light to dark brown).
♦ Evacuations that take more than 30 seconds or require pushing or grunting (they should be quick and easy).
♦ Discoloration in the bowel area of the iris (see the Chart on Iridology at the end of Chapter 7), especially tiny dark spots in this area. These spots indicate serious bowel pockets of long-lasting congestion, and possibly diverticulitis. The darker they are, the longer they have been there and the more serious the condition.
♦ Dark lines or spokes (radii solaris) protruding from the bowel area toward the circumference of the iris. Refer to the Chart on Iridology and note the area from the pupil to the autonomic nervous system; this is the area I am discussing.
♦ A history of taking antibiotics. They completely destroy the friendly intestinal flora.
♦ Lack of energy.
♦ Obesity.
♦ Unusual thinness.
♦ Poor complexion. Acne is a bowel problem. Teenagers who have acne need to cleanse as soon as possible, for their future health is at risk.

---

[74] As noted on page 20, the "diamond bullets" denote warning points.

Do you have any soreness in the colon area? Check the reflex points on the following chart. Soreness indicates bowel pockets and/or diverticulitis. Pinpointing the soreness may assist you in determining what area in the body may be affected. If you have problems in the areas indicated, you will now know the physical cause. And you can be sure that cleansing the intestines will be one of the most intelligent ways to rid yourself of those problems.

Ironically, those who need to cleanse the most, in many cases, seem least likely to do it, while those who least need it are often more inclined to do it. I suppose that people who unconsciously choose to suffer will avoid following programs that are effective.

Reflex Points of the Colon

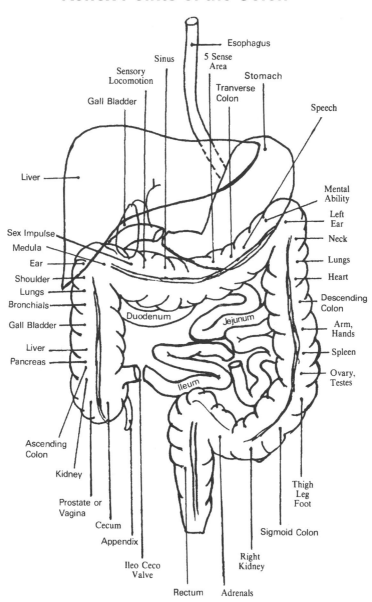

Esophagus

Sinus

5 Sense Area

Sensory Locomotion

Stomach

Gall Bladder

Tranverse Colon

Speech

Liver

Mental Ability

Left Ear

Sex Impulse

Neck

Medula

Ear

Lungs

Shoulder

Heart

Lungs

Descending Colon

Bronchials

Duodenum

Jejunum

Gall Bladder

Arm, Hands

Liver

Spleen

Pancreas

Ovary, Testes

Ileum

Ascending Colon

Kidney

Thigh Leg Foot

Prostate or Vagina

Cecum

Sigmoid Colon

Appendix

Ileo Ceco Valve

Right Kidney

Rectum

Adrenals

CHAPTER 9

THE POWERFUL ELEMENTS OF A SUPERB INTESTINAL CLEANSE

It has been more than 16 years since I first developed an intestinal cleanse, and over these many years I have experimented.[75] I have added one herb or enzyme and taken out another. I have perfected my formulas to such a degree that they actually dissolved the mucoid plaque into liquid before it was excreted from the body. Most people had superb results, but many people complained because they did not see the mucoid "ropes" coming out of them, as discussed in my writings. My consultants strongly recommended that I go back to one of my old formulas that produced the spectacular "ropes." I argued that I knew that people were better off with the more potent formula and so I continued with it. But complaints persisted and I finally gave in. So, with a few exceptions, people now see the "ropes" of mucoid plaque and they are happy, and so am I.

I doubt if anyone on this planet has experimented with cleansing as much as I have. It's been a passion all these years and still is. I've used hundreds of different enzymes, essential oils, homeopathic preparations, herbs – Chinese herbs, Ayurvedic herbs, and wild unknown herbs – the mind, visualization, and so forth. I have fine-tuned our cleansing program by first experimenting on myself, then on friends, animals, and even on my own mother. Everyone benefited. Close to a hundred thousand people have used my products, and I know what works and how to make it work even better. It can safely be used by just about anyone at any level of health and age. So now I am going to recommend a program that will work for anyone who uses it correctly.

Herbal Formulas

I apologize that I will not divulge the exact formulas. At one time I seriously considered doing just that, but I realized that are many who would misuse it. Anyone who knows me also knows that I demand the highest-quality herbs and ingredients available. With few exceptions, herbs should

---

[75] For more information on Dr. Anderson's most current research, see his Web Site (http://www.cleanse.net).

be either wildcrafted or organically grown. Most companies will not go that far, and they are making a terrible mistake. Herbs should be picked at certain times of the month, even at certain times of the day. They should be handled carefully, avoiding other herbs and pollutants. Herbs need to be dried under certain conditions, etc. Few are they who are willing to give this kind of effort. In the nutritional supplement and herb industry, like most other industries, there are those who care only about making money, and they will purchase the cheapest products available. And believe me, although health food stores are full of cheap and useless products, the junk in regular grocery and drug stores is often purely fraudulent.

I will give one example. One of the largest herbal product manufacturers in America advertises quality herbs. The company makes impressive claims about their products, which most of their customers believe. At one time I used to purchase herbs from them, but I kept having to send back many of their products; stating that they must have made some mistakes in their processing, for the products were only as good as worthless. Finally I realized that these were their standards, and then I stopped buying from them. Later, I was deeply involved with the purchasing of herbs on the "inner market" and I discovered what herbal suppliers thought about this company. One man put it this way: "If a supplier of herbs has a shipment of very poor grade and poor quality of herbs, which no one else will buy, every supplier can tell you that X company will buy it, if the price is right." So knowing what goes on out there in the so-called "real world," I decided to keep my formulas to myself, and keep an eye on the products that I recommend. Though it is difficult to be perfect, we always work for the highest level of quality possible.

Two Herbal Formulas – Keys to My Cleansing Program

Both these formulas contain specific herbs that caused the tremendous cleansing I experienced from eating raw, fresh herbs in our special meadow. They also contain other herbs that enhance other desirable effects necessary for maximum and safe cleansing. Each formula is needed to enhance the other and achieve the desired effect.

Formula 1 has the ability to increase peristalsis, and it is important to know how to use it properly. Formula 2 contains herbs that enhance Formula 1. It is an exceptional herbal nutritional formula that supports the body in the cleansing process and also enhances the effectiveness of Formula 1.

These two formulas are the heart of the program. If we used nothing else but these two formulas, the program would work, but it works far better if we use other products along with it.

Other Items Needed for the Cleanse

Sixteen-Ounce Shaker Container

This is used to make the "Psyllium Shake." Any container with a tight lid will do fine.

Enema or Colema Equipment

Enemas are one of the greatest inventions. They should be used for the deep phases of our program. A colema board is also recommended. But nothing works better than a colonic.

Psyllium Husk Powder

Psyllium husk *powder* should not be confused with psyllium *seed* or psyllium husk *whole*. For cleansing the intestines, you will need at least twice as much psyllium husk whole as you would with psyllium husk powder. And psyllium seed is practically useless.

When I first made our cleansing program available to the public, I did not use psyllium or bentonite. I used only the herbs. Back than, the majority of people who used our program were vegetarians. But, after about two years, more and more meat eaters were using it, and of course they were much more toxic than the vegetarians. Then we began receiving a large number of phone calls from people complaining of headaches, nausea, tiredness, and other cleansing reactions. I quickly realized that these people were highly toxic and the toxins were not being removed quickly enough, so of course cleansing reactions resulted. So I added psyllium and bentonite to our program, and that solved most of those complaints.

Psyllium, when used with liquid bentonite and other liquids, produces a mass of soft jelly-like substance. It gently but firmly scrapes the intestinal canal, acting like a broom and sweeping clean any *loosened* substance. Using bentonite with psyllium increases the effectiveness of the toxin-gathering mass by about 10 times.

A word of caution concerning psyllium: There are generally two versions of psyllium available to the public today. Both come from India. And, herbs originating in India typically carry high levels of contamination from either pathogenic bacteria and/or protozoan parasites. Some of these microorganisms have the potential to cause severe, long-lasting dis-ease and even death to people who have weakened their immune systems, and most people *have* weakened their immune systems. Therefore, the FDA and every credible herb supplier in America demand sterilization of all these herbs. Unfortunately most of the sterilization is done with radiation or ethylene trioxide, neither of which is acceptable to anyone who cares about health. Radiation leaves long-term, harmful nuclear partials, and ETO is simply another poison that can cause headaches, nausea, and possibly liver and kidney damage, and has been associated with development of cancer.[76] It is claimed the ETO evaporates from psyllium within a few days after treatment. This claim can be traced to manufacturers and is absolutely not true. Now, if I had to choose between radiation and ETO, which I do not have to do, I would use ETO; that's how bad radiation is. If I had to choose between ETO-treated psyllium, and non-treated psyllium from India, I would then choose ETO treated psyllium; **that's how dangerous non-treated psyllium from India is**. For it is much easier to eliminate ETO from the body than either radiation or the pathogenic bacteria or protozoan parasites from India or other foreign countries.

Fortunately, there is a better alternative. We searched diligently for a method to sterilize psyllium without leaving any unnatural residue *and we found it*! Our sterilization process uses a special steam heat procedure that eliminates all microorganisms and leaves the psyllium with a new and pleasantly clean taste. It works exactly as it always has, and without any possible chance of contamination – organic or inorganic.

Liquid Bentonite

Bentonite acts like a magnet or sponge, absorbing an amazing amount of toxic debris from the entire alimentary canal. It can absorb 40 times or more its own weight in toxins, bacteria, and parasites. **It should always be used with psyllium husk powder**. The only exception to this would be cases of food poisoning or severe vomiting. The combination of bentonite and psyllium works to pull loosened mucoid plaque from the

---

[76] From research conducted by the Seveso II Council Directive, See http://mahbsrv.jrc.it/Framework-Seveso2-Annex1.html See page 17 of 37 under Ethylene oxide: "Neurological disorders and even death after exposure have been reported. Probable human carcinogen."

walls of the intestinal tract. The loosened matter then adheres to the bulk of the psyllium, allowing a quick exit from the body.

Some people are concerned about the aluminum in bentonite. Yes, it does have aluminum; however, bentonite has a negative electrical charge, which is exactly the same charge that our epithelium cells of the gut have. Like the polar opposites of two magnets repelling one another, the cells of our bowels absolutely repel the bentonite from entering the inner sanctum of our bodies. This means that you never need to be concerned about absorbing anything that is in bentonite.

I have probably set the world's record in the consumption of bentonite. Oftentimes I still use it every day, for weeks at a time. Many times I have swallowed four (4) ounces at a time. I have no indication of aluminum poisoning, and hair analysis has never indicated any abnormal levels of aluminum in my body. Not long ago I passed my 58th birthday, and I am more alive than ever. I managed to break my arm skiing recently, but it healed in four weeks and I am once again back on the ski slope. The summer before last, I experienced the longest and most difficult backpack trip of my life. Today I can probably do anything that I have ever been able to do in my youth, and as I write this, my mind is clearer than it was last year, and my eyesight has also improved over the year before.

I think it is a sad mistake for people to be afraid of consuming bentonite. The Indians used it for centuries – and I may also use it for centuries!

How To Use Bentonite

Always use bentonite in liquid form. Using it as a powder can cause serious problems, and you might not realize it until long after the problems develop. In a dry form it could accumulate in the bowel and cause serious blockage to such a degree that surgery may be necessary to remove it. But **in a hydrated form, it does not cause any problem that I have seen and I know of tens of thousands of people who have used it**. One must not be fooled by cheap and ineffective products. Pure, distilled water and a high-speed hydrator are necessary to properly amalgamate bentonite into the proper hydrated form. A quality-hydrated **bentonite should be so viscid** that you may need to squeeze it out of the bottle.

Extra-thick bentonite not only means that you are getting your money's worth, but also that you can also use it for many other things. Bentonite is so useful that I have it in my first aid kit and even take it backpacking for weeks at a time. It draws and attracts toxins, mucus, and inflammation right out of your body. If a yellowjacket or bee stings you, put a dab of hydrated bentonite on it and the pain will disappear within a second or two. Put it on pimples and they dry up faster than with any medication. Put it on boils and the clay sucks the infection out in record time. Take a bath in it and poisons are pulled out of the skin. Ever banged a knee or elbow and had it become painfully swollen? Just place a thick bentonite poultice on the injury and the swelling and pain will be reduced in less than half the time it would take with anything else. It will even remove slivers and, help heal poison ivy as well as many other skin rashes. Bentonite sucks out inorganic minerals, drugs, and, to a certain degree, heavy metals. The moment it touches *E. coli* or some other pathogenic bacteria, or *Entamoeba histolytica,* those microorganisms are history. Too bad that the those AIDS patients who died from *E. histolytica* didn't know about cleansing and the power of bentonite. Bentonite will suck all those organisms it contacts, right into itself and will escort them right out of the body. Many times I have used bentonite after acquiring food poisoning from eating in a restaurant. I stir approximately 3 ounces in a glass of water and gulp it down. By the next morning there is no sign of a problem.

When using bentonite, **avoid any nutritional or herb supplement** *within a one-hour period*, for the bentonite will absorb the supplement. Even when used with psyllium, the bentonite will absorb anything of nutritional value, such as herbs, bacteria, and vitamins, as well as toxins, pathogenic bacteria, and parasites. It will also absorb acids, such as hydrochloric acid in the stomach. So be sure to wait one hour after drinking a psyllium-bentonite shake before consuming anything nutritious.

Bentonite is one of the volcanic ashes. It is not a drug or chemical composition made in a laboratory. It is a substance made by Mother Earth. Bentonite in ages past was blown into the sky by volcanic action, which sifted down to help impregnate the soil with its 25 to 35 trace minerals. Bentonite is good nutrition for plants, but not for humans, for we cannot assimilate it, nor do we want to, for the minerals are inorganic.

Though bentonite in a liquid form has been used internally by the American Indians for hundreds of years to help detoxify their bowels, I recommend that when using it internally, you *always* use it with psyllium. **The reason for this is that some people fear that bentonite could get stuck somewhere in the gut.** We do not know for certain if this has ever occurred with anyone, but just to be safe, I suggest using it with psyllium. The only exception may be for those who have acquired a bad case of food poisoning.

Purified Water

Purity is essential. Never drink, take a shower in, or swim in water with **chlorine or fluoride, for both are deadly poisons! Chlorine** was used in World War I as one of the agents in gas warfare. It is an extremely virulent poison. Even in minute concentrations, it is very toxic. That's why it is used in water, to kill bacteria and parasites. I have five clinical studies proving without doubt that chlorine from drinking water has caused several different types of cancer. Now if chlorine will cause cancer, consider what else it might be doing that is yet unknown to us. So, avoid it "like the plague."

Sodium Fluoride

This is a waste product from aluminum milling companies that has quietly and profitably been recycled into the bodies and brains of millions of Americans: *sodium* fluoride. The popularized concept that *sodium* fluoride is good for teeth is fraudulent – a dangerous lie. It has now been proven that it **does nothing to prevent tooth decay.**[77] **It is *calcium* fluoride, not *sodium* fluoride, which is good for the teeth**. Do our government decision makers know this? Perhaps some are not fully or accurately informed, but it is the responsibility of lawmakers to know the facts before they legislate. Certainly there would be major efforts by certain lobbyists to obscure the dangers fluoride poses. And even those who may be fully informed are no different than those in any other imperfect government in any other country. Money and power often, or in many cases, usually, speak louder than conscience. ***Sodium* fluoride in tap water actually increases tooth brittleness, likelihood of breakage, discoloration and periodontal bone loss.**[78] And since its use in cities, there has been **an increase in the number of mongoloid children born,**[79] **and in Alzheimer's** dis-ease.[80, 81]

---

[77] *Fluoride: The Aging Factor*, (Delaware, OH: Health Action Press, 1993). Chapter 14, pg. 114-132.

[78] C. C. Bass, "Neglect of Prevention of Dental Disease," *Journal of the Louisiana State Medical Society*, 1968; January; Vol. 120/Issue 1, pg. 30-35.

[79] Ionel Rappaport, "Second Study on Down's Syndrome and Fluoridated Areas," *Bulletin of the Academy of National Medicine, Paris*, 1959; Vol. 140, pg. 529-531.

[80] See the reference "Adverse Health Effects" at the Web Site (http://www.bruha.com/fluoride/html/adverse_health_effects.htm)

Sodium fluoride is a deadly poison that is used to kill rats by destroying the digestive system. **Sodium fluoride is a deadly heavy metal and is even more poisonous then lead.** Like so many other harmful substances, I believe the FDA allows it in our water because of the choices of key people who hold money and power. Adolf Hitler[82] and Communist Russia put *sodium* fluoride their water systems because it was thought that **sodium fluoride altered parts of the brain, which made people more susceptible to suggestion.** Clinical evidence may not be conclusive on this, but then even a suspicion along these lines would raise serious questions as to why our government demands the use of fluoride in city water, when evidence clearly indicates now that it does not solve dental problems and actually causes illness? So, the next question is: Why do you suppose anyone would want to make the public susceptible to suggestion?

If your city has fluoride in its water system, you will need to use distilled water, not just purified water. RO systems and filters cannot remove fluoride, and therefore you may need to either use distilled water or purchase pure water from out of town. Some people have stated that distilled water pulls minerals out of the body and therefore should not be used; the truth is that it can only remove inorganic minerals from the body, and that is exactly what we want it to do. The body cannot use inorganic minerals, and they can accumulate to cause congestion in our arteries, etc., so it strengthens the body to remove them. Organic minerals become part of our tissue, for they have been chelated to a protein molecule, and distilled water cannot attract organic minerals. The only problem with distilled water is that its life force is lost. But you can replace it by adding some freshly squeezed lemon, lime, or orange juice to it. But on the other hand, there is no life force in reservoirs or in most well water. Life force in water is found only in swiftly moving streams.

---

and, J. A. Varner, et al, "Chronic Aluminum Fluoride Administration: II. Selected Histological Observations," *Neuroscience Research Communications,* 1993; Vol. 3, No. 2, pg. 99-104; and M. Chase, "Rat Studies Link Brain Cell Damage with Aluminum and Fluoride in Water," *Wall Street Journal*, 1992; October 28.

[81] For more in-depth information on fluoride poisoing, see the book by Dr. John Yiamouyiannis, *Fluoride: The Aging Factor*, (Delaware, OH: Health Action Press, 1993). ISBN: 0-913571-03-2.

[82] Dr. Hans Moolenburgh, *Fluoride: The Freedom Flight,* Available only in German. May request from the National Library of Medicine through your local library.

Fruit Juice

Ideally, drink juice only fresh and *organically grown*. Make your own juice using apples, peaches, watermelons, cantaloupes, carrots, etc. Apples are still probably the best, but using berries, grapes, grapefruits, oranges, and, occasionally, pineapples are also fine. Second choice is to buy juice from stores that carry fresh, organic juice. Third choice is only for those who cannot do either of the above: They should at least purchase organically grown pasteurized fruit juice, which is readily available at any health food store.

Never drink juice from an average supermarket, for you can be absolutely certain that you will receive traces of poisonous pesticides, fertilizer residue, and herbicides, along with nutritionally deficient food values and, possibly, genetically modified substances, etc. Never, ever, drink juice that contains any added sugar, corn syrup, fructose, or any unnatural ingredients.

Use orange juice (and other citrus juices) only if you've been on the Cleanse several times and have never had a calcium problem. Orange is so cleansing that it can cause rapid elimination of toxic waste, making it difficult for the body to handle. Orange juice tends to extract calcium out of muscle, causing cramping, especially in the toes. Those who have weak kidneys should also avoid all citrus juices.

Anyone who has a **yeast infection, such as *Candida albicans*, or anyone who does not tolerate sugars, should use just plain water to mix with the psyllium shake.** They may also need to avoid carrot juice. I made a special psyllium mix for those with yeast infections; it contains specific herbs that help one with sugar problems and give a more pleasing taste to the psyllium. Some of us think that it tastes better than regular psyllium; it also helps balance the pH in the intestines.

Probiotics

The proper bacteria in the gut are essential for health. Few people realize just how important they are. In a healthy body, the total number of bacteria outnumbers man's own cells. Their total weight is comparable to that of the liver and they comprise close to 500 different strains. A perfect combination is required for health. Lack of certain bacteria could cause severe imbalances, and the abundance of certain species can also cause severe metabolic disturbances, along with vitamin B and amino acid deficiencies. Due to the *unnatural* lifestyles of most people, they have drastically altered their normal intestinal bacterial flora. This may cause a chain reaction of digestive disturbances, assimilation problems, liver weakness and deficiencies, which can contribute towards a gradual and consistent decline of health and towards the development of chronic and degenerative dis-ease.

Many people have used various acidophilus products with temporary success, only to later find that they had merely exchanged one set of problems for another. However, few have realized this because it is so difficult to trace symptoms back to the cause. Most bacteria formulas (Probiotics) contain a predominance of acid-producing bacteria (*Lactobacillus acidophilus* etc.), which are highly beneficial under various pathogenic conditions. I have a powerful probiotic containing this bacteria that works just as well as bentonite does for food poisoning. I always have it on hand, even when I'm traveling. It's amazing how many times I've given it to someone who had a sore throat or food poisoning and saw the problem vanish, usually overnight.

However, **when used for long periods of time, *Lactobacillus* bacteria can contribute towards ill health**. As I said above, I have two clinical studies in my possession that reveal a case of metabolic acidosis, a death-threatening, over-acid condition that was triggered by consuming *Lactobacillus* tablets and/or milk and yogurt. What are we doing to future metabolic functions when we saturate our bowels with acid-forming bacteria? *Acidophilus* bacteria, for an example, produce acids consisting of a pH of 3.9 to 4.5. This acid environment is in opposition to the normal bowel secretions of 7.5 to 8.9 pH. Not only that, but the digestive enzymes in the bowel can only function at a pH above a 7.0.

This is not to say that *Lactobacillus* do not have a place for human use, for they certainly have their place. As I noted above, studies have shown that these friendly bacteria serve an important role in the removal of pathogens, and in certain areas of the bowel. The main point is that *Lactobacillus* **should not be the predominant specie** in our gut.

Studies indicate that *Bifidobacterium infantis* is the predominant bacteria in the feces of breast-fed infants. This is the first bacterium that young, healthy infants receive from breast milk, and may be the most essential and core bacteria for the human gut. Other *Bifidobacterium,* such as *B. longum,* which is closely related to *B. infantis* and is found in both healthy children and adults, and *B. bifidum,* which is found in healthy adults, are probably the most natural and essential bacteria for man. These bacteria generate a pH between 6.5 and 7.0, which is much more beneficial for a healthy human bowel then the lactic-acid-producing ***Lactobacillus*** **that creates 3.9 to 4.5 pH**. Other beneficial bacteria begin to die off at a pH near 4.5, the upper limit of the pH normally produced by *Lactobacillus* *acidophilus.* As required, *Bifidobacterium* species are also known to produce large amounts of amino acids and other nutritious elements, including vitamins. Clinical studies have shown that out of all the other *Bifidobacterium* strains tested, both *B. Infantis* and *B. breve* were most effective in repelling *E. Coli* and *Salmonella,* and their toxins.

Friendly intestinal bacteria are essential to good health. Most **raw foods, especially those with chlorophyll, feed the friendly bacteria. Cooked and processed foods feed the harmful bacteria.** Undigested foods also feed pathogenic bacteria. The whole body must be in balance in order to have good health. When the bowel is out of balance, it becomes essential to take supplements of friendly bacteria. It is also critical to take *Bifidobacterium* after any use of antibiotics. Friendly bacteria are needed to help with the following:[83]

- Reduce cholesterol in the blood
- Produce certain digestive enzymes that help to digest proteins, carbohydrates, and fats
- Help control the acid-alkaline levels (pH) in the intestines
- Reduce unhealthy bacteria and yeast in the intestinal tract
- Reduce high blood pressure
- Detoxify poisonous material in the diet
- Assist the immune system
- Help with elimination of ailments such as colon irritation, constipation, diarrhea, irritable bowel syndrome, and acne
- Manufacture and assimilate B-Complex vitamins, especially vitamin B-12
- Produce natural anti-bacterial agents (antibiotics) which inhibit 23 known pathogens
- Produce cancer-suppressing compounds
- Detoxify hazardous chemicals added to foods and drugs
- Help calcium assimilation
- Help eliminate bad breath and gas.

---

[83] The "box bullets" indicate informational points.

The Most Dangerous Enemies of the Friendly Bacteria in Order of Importance[84]

> ♦ Drugs – especially antibiotics, since one dose can eliminate all friendly bacteria
> ♦ Alcohol – destroys friendly bacteria and enzymes, not to mention actual cells
> ♦ Pasteurized dairy products are gourmet meals for pathogens which destroy the good bacteria
> ♦ Cooked meat – it feeds the bacillus *E. coli* and other pathogens
> ♦ Bread – especially white flour or any wheat products that were baked in an oven (wheat is only good in its raw, sprouted state)
> ♦ White sugar – chocolate, cakes, pies, cookies, pop, catsup, etc.
> ♦ Fried foods – *e.g.* potato chips, French fries, and anything fried in oil
> ♦ Acid-forming foods, when overused
> ♦ Processed foods, such as pasta; all the food in packages

In conjuction with my good friend Dr. Khem Shahani, (Ph.D.), at the University of Nebraska, I have developed two probiotics. One is an extremely acid-producing bacteria and the other is only slightly acid-producing (6.5 to 7.0 pH). We use the strong acid-producer for the sole purpose of eliminating pathogenic microorganisms. And I am amazed at its efficiency. With food poisoning, for example, it is unequaled. It also eliminates most sore throats, that is, if the soreness is "germ"-related. I have not found anything that eliminates athlete's foot as effectively as this formula does: just sprinkle about one-eighth (1/8) of a teaspoon in your socks and wear the socks. This shows that it works against fungus, and it works fast. It is so potent that I caution people to not take more than one-quarter (1/4) of a teaspoon, except in the case of an emergency, such as in food poisoning, and then no more than one-half (1/2) a teaspoon taken three to five (3-5) times daily. Seldom will we need to take it for more than three or four (3-4) days. The only exception to this is when dealing with *long-term* yeast or bacteria infections. There are many places for pathogens to hide in the bowel, so under extreme conditions we may need to continue with this formula for 30 days and possibly longer, and ideally also be using

---

[84] As noted on page 20, the "diamond bullets" indicate warning points.

the Cleanse – a powerful, complete intestinal cleansing program, not just a colon cleanse.

I have made every attempt to clarify the need to follow the use of acid-producing bacteria with the less acid-producing formula. I cannot emphasize this enough. We also use this probiotic during and after cleansing and fasting. I used to recommend taking rectal implants to assure re-establishment of friendly bacteria. But with this new formula, that is no longer necessary. This formula is so effective that we can achieve a full implant, orally, within a few days. I recommend a week of use just to be certain, but usually a person can implant in 24 to 36 hours. Of course there are exceptions. Some people have a long-term acid environment, pathogenic yeasts and/or parasites that kill off every attempt to implant. And these people need to keep cleansing and keep using the probiotic formula that is only slightly acid-producing.

The Options

Ultimate Food Chlorophyll Concentrate

This is not the name of one of my most favorite super-herbal formulas, but it does describe this very beneficial formula. When people cleanse, they need to have a full spectrum of vital nutrients to nourish the body. **It is not wise to force the body into deep cleansing when it is deficient in the elements it needs to use for the process.** But people are doing this all the time, and these people are the ones who get into trouble.

A short time ago a member of my staff came in with a huge grin on his face and explained some of the results he had with the testing of this formula. He had asked a number of people to test the formula upon awakening in the morning. His sister and sister-in-law were the first to give him their results. He explained that both these ladies were "classic meat-eating, beer-drinking people trying to survive on the SAD (Standard American Diet.)" They had always resisted cleansing and other good health advice, but were willing to participate in this experiment for a week. After a few days, one of them developed a light headache which lasted for three days, and after that she felt better and had more energy. The eighth day came and this same lady concluded her experiment and went about her normal routine. However, within a few days, she noticed that her alertness and energy were down, and her sense of well-being had declined back to her prior, 'normal' levels. Then it hit her. This formula had indeed made her feel better, and she immediately arranged to continue her "experiment." She had not realized just how bad she had been feeling, but after feeling so much better, she then could see the contrast clearly.

His sister-in-law was of the same self-destructive disposition, being a heavy meat eater, coffee drinker, alcohol drinker, and consumer of the typical SAD (Standard American Diet). At the age of 38, she should not have been run down, but after consuming this product for a week, she was changed, for, in her own words, "it was like having two cups of coffee without the harmful side effects."

We were all happy that they felt better, but **I was saddened to more fully realize how depleted the average person has become, and to remember that this depletion always brings extraordinarily toxic accumulations.** It was good that these people did not jump into cleansing without preparation, for they were so depleted that they would probably have had severe cleansing reactions and would not have achieved the full benefits.

When people experience cleansing reactions and/or feel better simply by taking a supplement, it means they were seriously depleted. It shows that on a daily basis they were not receiving the nutrition they needed to maintain good health. It means that they have been on the road to serious dis-ease, **for if we fail to give our bodies the full spectrum of nutrients they need, dis-ease is imminent.** There is no nutritional supplement that will cause a healthy person to feel better, **if they already have everything a supplement can offer.**

As you can see, this formula could be highly beneficial to people who want the benefits of cleansing, and have failed to take good care of themselves. For these people, it is very important that they build up their nutritional reserves prior to cleansing or fasting.

Organic Electrolyte Minerals

As you know, electrolytes are essential for life and health. Here is a subject that I have researched deeply. I was shocked to discover that most Americans are deficient in electrolytes. My research has shown that there are no organic electrolytes available on the market. Most people are unaware of the difference between minerals coming from the vegetable kingdom and minerals from rock. I developed two organic electrolyte formulas that I believe are the most effective electrolytes available.

One of our distributors is a professional athlete. Several years ago she had depleted herself of electrolytes to a serious degree. She had tried many different electrolyte formulas available in health food stores, but failed to regain her strength. However, shortly after using my organic formula, she not only regained her strength, but also went on to place very high in the Hawaiian Iron Man Triathlon.

Each year thousands of people make the climb to the top of Mt. Shasta, a 14,164-foot mountain. The average person in good shape will make the climb, starting at 8,000 feet, in about 10 hours. Those who can make it in around five hours are known to be in outstanding shape. Persons who can make the climb in less than three hours are considered almost super-human. And most all those who have made the climb are quick to tell you that by the time they returned to the 8,000-foot level, they were utterly exhausted. And to walk the last mile back to the car is almost unbearable to most people. It takes the average person days to recover.

A friend of mine, Robert Webb at the age of 40, entered the *Guinness World Book of Records* by setting the world's record in elevation gained in a 24-hour period. In 1997 he climbed Mt. Shasta five (5) times in 24 hours. The next year he climbed it six (6) times in less than 24 hours. That's 37,000 feet in elevation gain in 24 hours, all of which was above 8,000 feet! Not only that, but his average climbs that day were less than three hours. Will this record ever be broken?

Robert is a vegetarian and uses my program to keep his body clean and free of congestion. He also used my ultimate food chlorophyll concentrate to build his body and took one of my organic electrolyte formulas, before, during, and after the climb. I also had him take a special herbal tincture I formulated that significantly helps people in high elevations, and while traveling in airplanes.

Liquified Minerals

Here is a very popular formula, containing organic, chelated, colloidal, non-toxic minerals, which means the minerals are in a state wherein they are tiny enough to be absorbed quickly and easily through cell membranes. These minerals come from a prehistoric vegetable residue and have been used by millions of people since the 1930's. They are well-proven to be extremely valuable for those who have not been assimilating their foods properly or who have not been on a good, clean, nutritious diet. In terms of cleansing, these liquified minerals greatly assist the metabolic enzymes in their process of elimination; and in terms of better health and overcoming dis-ease, they assist the enzymes in healing and rebuilding the body.

Reports about uses of this formula have reached near-miracle levels. I've heard isolated reports of gray hair returning to its natural color,

113

and rashes, arthritis, cataracts, diabetes, and other problems vanishing after using these minerals for an extended period of time. At best these minerals supply the body with trace minerals that it needs. It can also be used externally on rashes, sores, and bites and is excellent for burns and for the complexion. This formula is considered by some doctors and nutritionists to be the most complete and effective combination of organic trace minerals ever put together. It includes more than 60 minerals. People need these organic minerals, and most people are not getting them.

Using liquified minerals before, during, and after the Cleanse makes for better cleansing. You don't need them to clean out the mucoid plaque, but they help the body and bowel function better. These minerals are not high in electrolytes, but they are high in trace minerals. They work slowly but surely, and it is suggested that you take them for about seven (7) weeks before you judge their effectiveness.

Beware of other liquified minerals formulas. Various companies have claimed to include the exact same minerals, added about four to eight times as much water to weaken the bitter taste, and then added sweeteners to it. Yes, these formulas taste better, but you pay 4 to 10 times more for the same amount of minerals. And to top it off, some of these products cost far more than the concentrated version. I was at a show one time where a liquified mineral product was being sold at a booth. I purchased a quart and proceeded to drink it straight out of the bottle. Within two hours I drank the entire quart and I had no reactions. If the product had been of any value, I would never have been able to drink even a quarter of the bottle in two hours, for it would have triggered massive diarrhea. Minerals are powerful and can invoke many responses within our bodies.

All minerals are extremely bitter, so I suggest that you dilute them with either fresh citrus or grape juice. Prune juice works well to disguise the bitter taste, and pineapple juice is good too, but we cannot purchase quality pineapple juice. A dehydrated form of the liquified minerals formula may be preferred. Warning: The *liquified* minerals formula can produce a slight acidic effect. It should be used only when a person has a full alkaline reserve. In Chapter 11, I will explain how to test your alkaline reserve.

CHAPTER 10

IMPORTANT FACTS ABOUT AN OPTIMAL CLEANSING PROGRAM

"For just as the foolish physician studies dis-ease in order to bring about health, so the wise physician studies health in order to annihilate dis-ease, saying to his patients: 'Fulfill the condition of health, and dis-ease will fall away from you of its own accord.

Only the brave and the strong in spirit can hope to climb the precipitous mountainside to Divine knowledge, the weaker ones having to take the slower path, as any other course would inevitably result in their destruction."

– Dr. Rich Anderson

The Cleanse is Potent

I have investigated most of the colon cleanses on the market, and by that I mean I have used them myself. I have found that the program I subsequently was inspired to develop is, without a single exception, the most effective, powerful, and complete intestinal cleansing program available. I say this not only because of my research[85] and cleansing experience, but also because of the many hundreds of people who, after doing many other cleanses, finally did ours. With a united voice, they have proclaimed that our program was the most effective. The reason for this is simple. The two herbal preparations, Formulas 1 and 2, bring together unique combinations of herbs. Unlike most programs similar to it, this program cleanses the stomach and small intestine, as well as the colon. **Due to its unusual potency, it must be used wisely and with caution.**

A potent herbal cleansing program, be it for the bowels, liver, or any other organ or system, can cause cleansing reactions. Most companies

---

[85] For more information on Dr. Anderson's latest research see his Web Site (http://www.cleanse.net).

do not want to answer people's questions about cleansing reactions, as cleansing reactions can easily be misunderstood. By making sure their products are not very potent, these companies vastly diminish the likelihood that any of their customers will ever have to wonder what a cleansing reaction is! For the sake of providing a cleansing program that really works, I have been willing to provide assistance for people on the issue of cleansing reactions. This book includes a chapter on the topic, and I have written a separate booklet, "Dramatic Signs of Healing," which goes into depth on this matter. This information proves invaluable for anyone who is undertaking profound and effective internal cleansing such as my formulas facilitate.

Four Phases of Cleansing Adaptable to Individual Needs

For a cleanse to be effective and health nurturing, it must be geared to the level of strength and health available in the body. A deeper, more powerful cleanse releases old toxins very quickly; **only a body that has already achieved a significant level of strength and health can handle this degree of cleansing**. When one is weak or fighting illness at the outset of cleansing, the process must be taken more slowly, lest the body's ability to remove toxins be overwhelmed, resulting in increased but unnecessary stress, and extreme cleansing reactions. Hence, I have developed four stages of cleansing, which can be alternated, as needed, to meet individual needs. I call these the four phases:

- ❑ Mildest Phase, with 2-1/2 meals daily
- ❑ Gentle Phase, with 2 meals daily
- ❑ Power Phase, with 1 meal daily
- ❑ Master Phase, with juices only.

The Most Important Rule in Using the Phases

During all four phases, **we should always feel relatively good**. We can expect a few mild cleansing reactions, but it is no longer necessary to "tough it out." Common cleansing reactions include headaches, aching muscles or joints, sweating, rashes, bad breath, sleepiness, weakness, dizziness when standing, and, occasionally, nausea. When cleansing reactions occur, it is because the body cannot remove the toxins and acids as fast as they are being released from storage into circulation. To reduce cleansing reactions, we simply need to assist our elimination organs:

- ❑ First take a colonic or enema (a colonic is better).
- ❑ If that doesn't help, take a *coffee* colonic or enema.[86]
- ❑ If that doesn't help, it is best to go back to an earlier phase until feeling good again. Eating heavier foods, as indicated below, will slow the cleanse process and allow the elimination organs to catch up on handling any back-up of toxins.
- ❑ Then, progress again through the phases at a comfortable pace. Allowing ourselves the "luxury" of feeling bad can be hard on the liver, kidneys, heart, and brain, and is simply not necessary. I no longer recommend it.

Alternating Between Phases

One of the advantages of using this four-phase program is that we can control our cleansing reactions and also accommodate our social life, simply by alternating between the four phases. In other words, we can switch back and forth from one to the other, as needed. **It is in this way that we can keep cleansing reactions to a minimum, boost our energy when needed, and keep on feeling good while cleansing**. The milder phases are great for those who just do not have the will power to do the full Cleanse (no meals), who have to work full-time, have an exceptionally heavy work schedule, have social obligations, have a great amount of toxicity, or have energy problems. But remember this: Most people who do our cleansing program **work full-time while cleansing.** Alternating between phases makes it possible for a person to remain in top condition while cleansing, so that a normal work schedule is easy to maintain.

Example: let's say a person begins with the Gentle Phase (two meals per day) for four weeks, then spends a few days on the Power Phase (one meal per day), and then progresses on to the Master Phase of the Cleanse. Three days into this final phase, he starts feeling weak, which affects his work. It is a good idea, then, for him to switch back to the Power Phase, eating one meal a day. Perhaps that perks him up, and the next day he goes back to the Master Phase. If not, it may be a good idea for him to stay on the Power Phase for a longer period, or even to go back to one of the gentler phases. **Eating meals slows down the cleansing, and the toxic flow is lessened.** By the weekend or on his days off work, he may feel OK to use the full cleanse again. Then Monday he can go back to one of the other phases again, if needed. It is good to be flexible.

---

[86] See Chapter 13: "How to Take an Enema."

Note: It takes between four and seven days before the herbs condition the mucoid plaque to release. Also, the action of the herbs has momentum; taking a break from the herb may require beginning all over again.

The Elderly, Weak, and Extremely Toxic: Those Who Cannot Pass the pH Tests

These people should always begin with the Mildest Phase. If they continue feeling OK after a week or so, and if they passed the pH tests, they may begin the Gentle Phase. However, they should be ready to alternate between the Gentle and Mildest Phases. The point is that, by switching from one phase to another, a person can control how he or she feels, continue obtaining maximum nutrition, and keep cleansing reactions to a minimum. **Those who do not pass the pH tests should not go beyond the mildest phase** until they have sufficiently boosted their electrolyte reserves so that they can pass the pH tests. To accomplish this, they should be sure to drink plenty of fresh, raw, organic vegetable juices and take natural electrolyte supplements made with vegetable juice concentrates, etc. I have designed one, which is available to supplement an ideal cleansing program. I have also designed another supplement to accomplish the same purpose for those who have sugar-related problems, such as diabetes, hypoglycemia, Candidiasis, etc.

Note: The real so-called "miracles" of cleansing usually occur while on the Master Phase – with no solid food for seven days. Almost everyone will have wonderful results on the lesser programs, but nothing works the "magic" as does the "Master Phase."

Four Phases of Cleansing

The Mildest Phase

This phase was developed to make cleansing possible for those who are significantly weak or toxic. I developed this program for my mother, not because of her age or because of her toxins, but because I did not believe that she had the will to go deeper, and I knew that she would not be able to pass the pH tests because she would not improve her diet. It worked; she had splendid results. It corrected so many problems for her that even I was surprised.

The pH tests are used to determine if a person has the necessary electrolyte reserves to safely accomplish cleansing. **If one cannot pass the**

pH tests, the Mildest is the only phase to use. While on this phase, the cleanser may continue to check pH to determine when it is wise to proceed on to the next phase. When using this phase, the cleanser takes two and one-half alkaline-forming meals each day, in addition to a regimen of cleansing herbs and shakes. This phase is very gentle on the body, and yet can be a very effective aid towards improving health and energy. Once cleansers have achieved a level of stability with this regimen, that is, they are able to maintain it without uncomfortable cleansing reactions and have passed the three parts of the pH test, they may safely progress on to the next phase of cleansing. **But, if cleansing reactions are experienced on this phase, the cleanser should**[87]:

❑ Increase intake of organic electrolyte minerals made from dehydrated vegetable juices[88] (which the body needs to remove toxins and acids).[89]

❑ Take a colonic or enemas if elimination is sluggish, and by that I mean less than three (3) voluminous bowel movements daily.

❑ Increase intake of the two (2) herbal formulas to achieve three to four (3-4) easy eliminations daily.

❑ Eat more foods that slow down the Cleanse process, such as potatoes.[90]

On this phase and the Gentle Phase, use colonics or enemas as needed. Many people do not need any colonics or enemas during these phases.

The Gentle Phase (Beginning)

Most persons should use this phase to begin their cleanse. Some people try to skip this phase, thinking they don't need it; this is a mistake. Even when your body is perfectly healthy, this phase is needed to give the herbs time to prepare and soften up mucoid plaque for most effective

---

[87] As noted on page 20, the "box bullets" indicate informational points.

[88] Dehydrated vegetable juices contain the most concentrated sources of organic electrolytes available.

[89] Many cleansing reactions are caused by acids being released from the body. The body needs to use electrolytes to safely remove these acids. When the body is deficient in electrolytes, and acids are being released, cleansing reactions can be severe.

[90] See the chart on Alkaline-forming and Acid-forming Foods in Appendix 1.

removal. Some persons will find plenty of challenge and reward in this phase alone, and choose to do only the Gentle Phase in their first cleanse or two. This phase involves eating two alkaline-forming meals per day, and all the fresh carrot/celery/beet[91] juice one desires, along with a complementary regimen of herbs and shakes. After a cleanser has reached a level of stability where he or she can maintain the Gentle Phase comfortably, with no cleansing reactions, then that person may safely progress on to the next, deeper phase of cleansing. If cleansing reactions should persist *during any phase of cleansing*, even after following the steps described under the Mildest Phase for handling cleansing reactions, the cleanser should return to a milder phase of cleansing to slow the Cleanse down and make it easier on the body. If a person has excessive cleansing reactions on the Mildest Phase, they may need to cease cleansing, and concentrate on building their alkaline reserve until it improves enough to handle cleansing better. Some persons with serious parasite infestation may need to cease the Cleanse and do my parasite program first, then return to the Cleanse. Once a person has been on the Gentle Phase for 3 weeks and is feeling good, he or she may go to either the Power or Master Phase.

Note: I recommend that you remain on the Gentle Phase for three (3) weeks if it is your first cleanse. The more toxins you can remove before going on to the Master Phase, the easier and more efficient the Master Phase will be. If it is your second cleanse, then you may do two (2) weeks of the Gentle Phase, and those experienced with the Master Phase who have few or no cleansing reactions should do at least one (1) week.

The Power Phase

This phase demands more commitment, strength and body vitality. Many people will use the Power Phase as a test to determine whether they are really ready to do the Master Phase. After being on the Power Phase for two (2) or three (3) days without cleansing reactions, then they know they are ready for the Master Phase. Some people may stay on the Power Phase longer if they choose. On the Power Phase, the cleanser takes one (1) alkaline-forming meal per day, and all the fresh juices desired, along with a complementary regimen of herbs and shakes. As the amount of solid food intake is decreased, the body is freed more and more from its usual digestive tasks, and can devote increased attention to its cleansing priorities.

---

[91] Those with significant sugar sensitivity should avoid all sweet juices, both fruit and vegetable. However, they may want to take other fresh organic vegetable juices, such as kale and other greens.

Note: While on the Power and Master Phases, urine pH tests are of no use, because the body will be removing so many acids that the tests will not reflect true electrolyte reserve levels. The saliva pH test may or may not be accurate, depending upon the acids in the mouth. The only reliable pH test during these phases is the lemon test.

The Master Phase

Truly, those who can complete this phase have greater mastery over their bodies than most people. During this final phase of cleansing, no meals are taken. A regular regimen of herbs and shakes are taken to help the body remove sometimes-astounding amounts of mucoid plaque. Fresh, organic fruit[92] and vegetable juices, as well as high-quality green super-herbal drinks, may be taken for additional nourishment during this phase, which typically lasts one (1) week. This phase is obviously the most challenging and the most rewarding. Cleansers who accomplish this phase of cleansing report stories of seemingly miraculous healing.

Fresh, Organic Juices and Water Essential for Health and Effective Cleansing

Drinking fresh juices from organically grown fruits and vegetables, on a daily basis, is one of the wisest and most effective things anyone can do to achieve and maintain good health. Organically grown foods have approximately 75% to 350% the nutritional and mineral value of commercially grown foods.[93] We need nutrition to be healthy; fresh juices supply concentrated levels of that nutrition. Not only that, but they are full of life force! I suggest reading additional books on juicing and fresh, organic juices.

As implied, one of the best aids to a powerful cleanse is the generous use of fresh, organic juices. They offer a concentrated source of live enzymes, as well as easily assimilated minerals and vitamins. These further prompt and strengthen the body's cleansing activity. **I encourage all those who cleanse to obtain a good juicer and make their own fresh,**

---

[92] Orange juice is not recommended while cleansing because it contains too much acid.

[93] John Boik, *Cancer & Natural Medicine*, (Princeton, MN: Oregon Medical Press, 1996), pg.146.

organic vegetable juices. Fruit juices are excellent, too. The citrus juices have the strongest cleansing effect, and should only be used with moderation (if at all) by those who have a high level of toxicity, and a tendency toward low pH, for citrus contains acids that can overtax electrolyte levels for some people. The only exception to my encouragement to use juices is that **those with sugar sensitivity[94] should avoid all sweet juices.** Fresh, organic juices are especially important during the final phase of cleansing when no solid food is taken.

Note: Will vegetable juices such as carrot juice slow the cleansing down? Yes, it will. However, I strongly recommend that you use the vegetable juices for at least the first few cleanses. Using the Master Phase with water only will speed up detoxification significantly. For most people, it will speed it up too much. In the past I did not recommend juices on this phase, but people are much more toxic than they were 10 years ago. Remember, America is becoming weaker with each generation. (I'm trying to help remedy this frightful trend, but I haven't had much help from the medical community.)

The more juices we drink, the less water we desire. However, even though you are drinking plenty of water while cleansing, it is important to drink at least an additional 64 ounces a day of pure, non-chlorinated and non-fluoride water (preferably distilled water that is stored in glass or especially high-grade plastic containers – not the standard supermarket-grade plastic container). It should be clean water from a well or spring; water purified with a solid carbon block or other high-quality unit, or distilled water. Many advocate distilled water for its added cleansing effects; it also helps extract inorganic minerals and toxic waste from the body.

Water is critical while cleansing because **without enough water, elimination is sluggish and cleansing reactions are increased.** On a hot summer day, the average-size person should drink about a gallon of water a day while cleansing; that is, about one ounce of water for each pound of body weight. On cooler days, at least 3 quarts of water are needed, but it is important to realize that **it is better to drink too much water than not enough.**

Note: If cleansing reactions occur, drink more water. Even if you are drinking extra water, it may not be enough. When cleansing reactions occur, you should drink enough water that you need to urinate once an hour, and maybe more.

---

[94] Includes those who are hypoglycemic, diabetic, and who have yeast infections, such as Candidiasis.

Super Results of the Final Phase

People doing our gentler cleansing regimen get wonderful results. They remove a great deal of toxicity from their bodies. **But, it is on the Master Phase of the full cleanse, with adequate preparation during the beginning phases, that people obtain the miraculous results.** There is something about going without food that has incredible transformative powers. It seems to work on all levels of our being: the mental, emotional, spiritual, and the physical.

On the physical level, **when we stop eating, our bodies scavenge the** *excess* **proteins that are responsible for many of our health problems.** This includes proteins that are **stored in our livers and kidneys, and even in our cells. Truly, these are the proteins that cause most of the dis-ease in this world.** Excess proteins not only acidify our bodies, because protein foods are acid-forming foods, but they create mucus and congestion. That is one of the reasons that our livers and kidneys malfunction. When we fast, the stored proteins are attacked by our bodies and degraded into amino acids,[95] then deaminated and oxidized, and used just as though we were still eating.[96] **We're similar to camels, except that instead of storing large amounts of water to save our lives, we store proteins, which are killing us.** Congestion is the primary cause of dis-ease on the physical level and **fasting removes congestion.** Proper fasting never attacks the proteins we need; only the ones we don't need. Imagine, removing all this excess protein and everything else that is clogging up our systems! Fasting is not starvation until it reaches a certain point, and that point is usually between 40 to 60 days of having nothing but water.

I have found that inharmonious thoughts and feelings are stored in many of the proteins that contribute towards dis-ease. This is why fasting can favorably alter consciousness – remove depression and habits of negative thinking.

---

[95] The composition of parasites and bacteria is mostly protein. Imagine on a long fast what might happen to these guys. Ahh, we have the picture now. So maybe this is why the greatest and most incredible individuals who ever walked the earth, fasted so many times. Fasting cleans up the body, mind, emotions, and spirit. However, in this day and age, we have exceptionally overpolluted bodies, which are saturated with large amounts of chemicals and drugs, and **we cannot fast like they used to without intelligent preparation.**

[96] Guyton, pg. 833.

Talk about relief! Many people have described radical shifts in consciousness – from worry and stress to bliss consciousness; from depression and despair to optimism and joy. As of the time of this writing, all persons I know of who accomplished our cleanse and had critically high blood pressure, found their blood pressure to be normal before they completed the Master Phase. There was only one exception to this – a man doing the Cleanse in the hospital. He had suffered greatly because of the equipment attached within him and because of having to eat hospital "food" (so-called!) Even so, his blood pressure improved by 50%. People with bone cancer pain (about the worst pain of all) found 75% of their pain gone within six days, and that was without coffee enemas.[97] We have many testimonies of people whose severe back pain disappeared, or was greatly diminished, before finishing the Cleanse. Hundreds of people have reported their pains disappearing while cleansing. What do you suppose is happening to our bodies when we get relief so quickly like this? The Cleanse simply removes congestion – congestion of the mind, spirit, and body.

How Long Do I Stay on the Cleanse?

An ideal cleanse program for the average person is suggested to last four weeks, with two and one-half weeks on the Gentle Phase, one-half week on the Power Phase, and one week to 10 days on the Master Phase. This guideline should be modified to meet individual body needs, according to how each person's body responds while cleansing. A person who is highly toxic needs to move more slowly, spending more time on the gentler phases, in preparation for accomplishing the Master Phase without serious cleansing reactions.

There are no instructions that can give all persons the perfect suggestions for their own unique conditions. **Each person is responsible for his or her own body. ALWAYS USE YOUR OWN INTUITION AND COMMON SENSE.** When on the two most gentle phases of our cleanse program, we can continue cleansing as long as we feel it is right for us. But **if it doesn't feel right, either stop or don't begin until it does**. Fear attracts that which you fear! Deep cleansing is not for those who are dominated by fear and apprehension.

---

[97] These persons used coffee colonics or enemas, along with the regular Cleanse program. Coffee colonics or enemas are noted for their ability to relieve pain.

124

Never Feel Hungry

Many people do not believe us when we say that while on the Cleanse you won't feel hungry. But, you will be so full of herbs and juices that you really won't. Some may still struggle with the desire to eat, nonetheless, because of old, old habits. The desire to eat, however, is not necessarily related to hunger.

People would be amazed how little food they really need. Most people eat about four times more food than they really need, and this causes problems. I love to eat, but I rarely eat more than two meals daily. However, I will snack on fruit if I get hungry. Going without food once in awhile helps to tone up the body, and gives it a chance to eliminate unwanted substances.

How Often Can I Cleanse?

For the enthusiast, every seven to ten weeks is recommended for the first year of using the full cleansing program, as long as the pH tests show adequate electrolyte levels. Most people receive terrific benefits cleansing once every six months. That is my recommendation for the average person.

Those who will not venture beyond the Mildest or Gentle Phases of the Cleanse may continue as long as it feels right to continue, and as long as good, nutritious eating habits are followed. However, I do recommend that you stop and give yourself a break for a week or so about once every six or seven weeks; and the longer one continues, the longer should be the breaks.

In two to three years many people could achieve a state of health that would absolutely delight them. This has been found to be true of people who are even in their 80's, and it certainly was for me. But once the mucoid plaque has been eliminated, you will find that you do not want to continue with intestinal cleansing. This is when water and juice fasting are needed to produce the greatest results.

My work in life has been research, and I research everything that offers potential for health improvement; but I have never found anything that deserved so much attention as an effective cleansing program, and I have never seen or heard about anything that brings people back to health as rapidly or effectively as this can. Nor have I found anything that even comes close, and many thousands will testify to this truth.

I find it almost unbelievable that there are so few doctors who have realized that de-clogging the system and giving the body natural, wholesome foods is the most logical treatment in overcoming dis-ease and establishing good health. It boggles my brain to think that doctors who should be experts in healing are so naïve, ignorant, and even stupid, to the point where they think that surgery, drugs, radiation, or even things that are helpful, (vitamins, proteins, superfoods, acupuncture, homeopathics, or some "super" chemical) will bring someone back to health while the person is still jam-packed to overflowing with mucus, toxins, acids, worms, etc.

I have also found that the few good products that actually do help people are much more effective after a person cleanses. So when we combine this program with the other alternative healing methods available (such as the helpful supplements and processes mentioned above) we increase the healing potential by many times. A thorough cleansing program will greatly enhance every other constructive healing method known and may very well make the difference between success or failure – and to some, life or death.

How Many Cleanses are Necessary to Be Completely Cleaned Out?

Every person is different. With me, it took about twelve cleanses; however, I did not have the advantages that are available now. For my first nine cleanses, I used other methods, which I call "mini-cleanses" (colon cleanses). On those cleanses I eliminated about 12 to 14 feet in seven days. Towards the end, after modifying them, I eventually was able to remove 28 feet in seven days; and when I finally developed our cleansing program, I removed more than 40 feet in seven days. **Dr. Jensen says that it sometimes takes several cleanses before some people can remove *any* mucoid plaque.** Fortunately that has not been the case with our program. The vast majority of people get results during their first cleanse if, of course, the instructions are followed.

Factors Affecting Long-Term Cleanse Results[98]

❑   Your overall current condition
❑   Your attitudes and subconscious patterns
❑   How closely you follow the cleansing instructions

---

[98] As noted on page 20, the "box bullets" indicate informational points.

- How well you eat between cleanses
- Which phases of the Cleanse you follow
- The condition of your liver

Motivation for Cleansing

Right now you may be thinking, "I'm not even sure I want to do one cleanse, let alone two or three a year." To you, my friend, let me simply encourage you to *try* it. Even if you only did a cleanse once a year, or just the Mildest Phase, you would be giving your body enormous relief, saving it from the tiresome task of spending all its energy digesting and protecting itself from the overload of proteins, acids, and toxic matter we thoughtlessly dump into it three times a day (this doesn't even include snacking and coffee breaks). How much is your health worth to you? This once-a-year vacation would give the body a chance to take a breather and devote its energy to healing itself. Besides, you may change your mind once you make it through the first time. The most important thing is to muster your courage and venture a first step into the unknown. But if you fear it, then don't even try it.

It's true, not everyone can do this. You will be distinguishing yourself from the majority of human beings who accept ill-health as a cruel twist of fate and unconsciously struggle blindly through life, or who have neither the wisdom nor the courage to remove causes of potential suffering and dis-ease. These do not take responsibility for their lives, have victimized themselves, and have become totally dependent upon doctors for their security. Not only will you be saved from their fate, but after you have completed your first cleanse, you won't be made of the "same old stuff" anymore, and not only will you know this from experience, but you will know it from the way you feel. You will be proud of yourself, and realize that **the stuff of which you now really are made *is* better than what you were made of before you accomplished the Cleanse!**

The Iris Reflects Health Improvement After Cleansing; Eye Color May Even Change

Some cleansers have reported significant changes in their iris, which reflected changes in their physical condition. Markings indicate congested or stressed areas, and when we cleanse deeply enough, we can lighten the dark areas. It is interesting to have a photo taken of your irises before cleansing, and again four weeks after completion of your cleanse.

My friend Jonni Sue Perlman's eyes changed dramatically after cleansing. They went from brown, like her mother's, to a beautiful greenish-hazel. When she started cleansing, she was, seemingly, already in excellent health. She did, and still does, exercise almost daily, and has been a vegetarian for more than 20 years. So the strength of her body is capable of supporting rapid changes. At the time of this writing, another person has just written me, claiming that her irises had also radically changed color.

The Tongue

Many people notice that as they cleanse, their tongues turn whitish-gray and filmy, and the breath becomes more and more foul. This reflects what is happening inside the digestive canal. As they use the herbs and drink fresh juice, mucoid layers will soften, and so they may notice that the abdomen swells. As more and more mucoid layers are removed, the swelling goes down, the tongue gradually becomes clearer, and the breath improves. This is a good gauge as to how clean a person is becoming, **for when you are totally clean, the tongue will be shiny red** (just like a newborn baby's). **It will be free of all whiteness or film, and the breath will be sweet** (unless we eat onions, garlic, or dairy products). Even the bowel movements can become sweet smelling, though poor eating will cause odors to return. Let this be one of our goals: to have a pleasant fragrance throughout.

Identifying the Origin of the Mucoid Plaque[99]

The cleansing program that I have developed is far more than a colon cleanse. It can cleanse the entire gastrointestinal tract or alimentary canal – all the way from the tip of the tongue to the anus. Although the colon tends to accumulate thicker layers than do the other areas, the majority of what most people observe being expelled while cleansing is from the small intestine. Due to the way the intestinal wall is formed and because the mucoid was originally liquid and has been adhering to the walls of the intestines for so many years, the mucoid layers naturally take on the same shapes and creases as the areas where they were formed.

Most cleansers have seen these striations in their mucoid plaque, and you can also see them in the pictures provided in this book. Studying

---

[99] See photos of mucoid plaque in Chapter 3: "The Digestive System and the Creation of the Dreaded Mucoid Plaque," following the section, "What is Mucoid Plaque?"

the photos and reading the following descriptions may help you to identify the locality, or source, of your evacuations. This could be of interest if there were certain problems that you wanted to correct. When we can identify where the plaque came from, we may be able to determine if some of our problems are about to be flushed down the toilet. In that case, hurrah!

Descriptions of Plaque from Different Portions of the Digestive Tract

When the plaque comes from the **stomach**, it is eliminated as roundish globs of rubbery mucus. This is rare to see. Plaque in the stomach could inhibit the production of hydrochloric acid, and of course protein digestion would be inefficient.

The **duodenum** is the first portion of the intestine, located just below the stomach. It's about 10 inches in length, and is one of the most important areas in the alimentary canal. It is here that digestive juices from the gallbladder and pancreas enter the intestines. It is also in the duodenum that important digestive enzymatic activities should occur to prepare food for proper digestion. Contrary to other areas of the bowel, the striations or folds of the duodenum are multi-directional, flowing out from and around small circles, which reveal the locations of pancreatic and bile ducts. Mucoid plaque in this area could severely inhibit digestion by interfering with pancreatic and bile juices. It could also contribute towards pancreatic and gallbladder problems, ulcers of the duodenum, and an acid bowel.

The **jejunum** is located just below the duodenum. About eight and one-half feet long, here the special cells of the intestinal wall secrete various chemicals and enzymes to be combined with gallbladder and pancreatic juices. In this manner, the small intestine controls the digestive process. A large proportion of nutrients are assimilated here. The folds in the jejunum are closely packed, and run in one direction. This is where the Peyer's patches are located. The Peyer's patches may have a direct effect upon the thyroid. If mucoid plaque were in the Peyer's patches area, then by nerve reflex, the thyroid could be affected. Elimination of plaque from that area is a good clue that digestion and thyroid may improve.

The **upper ileum** is found just below the jejunum. Combined with the lower ileum, it accounts for about 12 feet of the length of the small intestine; assimilation is its major function. The folds are shallower and fade away as it approaches the colon. The striations actually disappear in the lower ileum, so the plaque is smooth and shiny.

The colon has no striations, but does have definite overlapping circular rings. This is caused by its accordion-like haustrations. Thick mucoid plaque in the colon simply indicates toxicity, not only in the colon, but also in the entire body. It is in the colon where bowel pockets (pockets of extreme toxicity) are most common and bowel pockets are the precursors to diverticula. The Merck Manual says that diverticula are present in 30 to 40% of persons over age 50, and their incidence increases with each subsequent decade of life. It also notes that among those who live long enough, diverticula are present in close to 100% of the American people. Of course this does not include people who cleanse themselves, nor most vegetarians, or those who do not eat the Standard American Diet (SAD).

Psyllium or Mucoid Plaque?

Many have questioned whether they were indeed eliminating the mucoid plaque or just the psyllium. Here is how to tell: The psyllium, after passing through the body, is *never* evenly formed, never smooth, and never consistent in size or shape. It never has even lumps, creases, overlaps, smoothness, or striations, and it is never shiny like the plaque usually is.

If you look carefully at the psyllium after it has passed through the bowel, and use a magnifying glass, you will see that it looks like miniature pollywog eggs. It has very tiny, egg-like centers with a jelly-type substance surrounding it – about one sixty-fourth (1/64) of an inch in size. You have to carefully scrutinize to see it clearly, but it's there. If you don't see it, then you are looking at something else. However, the mucoid plaque may not always have (though it usually has *some*) striations, smoothness, overlaps, and creases. But it never looks like psyllium. The plaque is usually shiny and often looks like thin or thick pieces of leather or rubber.

During the Cleanse, the color of psyllium generally remains the same coming out as it was going in. This is particularly true while on the Power and Master Phases.

Another way to identify plaque is to slice the eliminated material and examine it. If the mass on the inside is different from that on the outside, either in color or texture, then you know for sure that you have removed a mucoid layer.[100] Sometimes mucoid plaque comes out without the psyllium medium, but you will have no trouble identifying these pieces.

---

[100] The only exception to this statement is that when we're on the intermediate or one of the beginning phases and still eliminating food, the inner part may be regular feces.

No Mucoid Plaque!

Several years ago, I met the first person who claimed that no mucoid plaque came out of him during the Cleanse. I asked him one question after another to find out if he, like many other people, simply didn't know how to identify mucoid plaque. Yes, he had followed the instructions perfectly. Indeed, his description of what he eliminated did sound like psyllium. It turns out this man had been raised as a vegetarian from birth, on a farm in Germany, miles from the nearest city. They ate foods almost entirely from their own farm and most of it was raw. **He had never been sick a day in his life**. He actually was brought up under what I would call ideal conditions. I have never seen anyone else like him. His skin looked as though he was from another planet. It was 100% free of blemishs and wrinkles, smooth, soft, and radiant. His skin and hair glowed to such a degree that he looked a little unusual; and his skin appeared almost transparent. He was extremely harmonious, confident, and happy, as he revealed in his mannerisms. I couldn't help but envy him a bit. I asked him if he had received any benefits from the Cleanse. He said that during the Cleanse he felt spiritually elevated, but he gained no physical benefits that he could tell. He felt perfect before the Cleanse and felt perfect after the Cleanse. When you're perfect, you can't get better.

If Only Liquids or Small Pieces are Removed

Some people expel only small pieces, from microscopic to four or five inches. Generally they look like little pieces of leather. Some of these people have complained that they not eliminating anything at all! For example, one lady called me from Phoenix, to tell me that she had been cleansing for ten days and nothing had been eliminated. That was 30 psyllium shakes, with nothing coming out! I knew that something was wrong, because if nothing was being removed, then by now she must be the size of a rhinoceros and just as mean. Finally, she admitted that black liquids were coming out. So the next question was, how many herbs was she taking? She was taking tablets, 50 of each herbal formula a day, and the liquids were black. I explained to her that the herbs were pulverizing and liquefying the mucoid plaque. She kept waiting to see big chunks being removed, and they were, but in liquid form. Unfortunately, we can't measure how much comes out that way, but I believe it's considerable.

One doctor gave me a full, day-by-day report of his cleanse. He took 40 tablets of my herbal formula a day, which caused him to eliminate the plaque in liquid form, but he felt he was getting rid of more that way and was not concerned about cutting back on the herbs and watching for the big pieces. One advantage to this method is that you don't need to take colonics or enemas, as there will likely be several eliminations a day. However, it is important to remember that each person is unique, and responses to the same amounts of herbs may vary widely. Not only that, **but our bodies change as we cleanse, and our needs change**.

Cleansing and Candida

Those who have Candidiasis and are planning to do our cleanse program should have very good results if they follow the guidelines below and use the friendly bacteria (probiotic) supplements correctly. However, those with advanced cases of Candida are strongly advised to secure the help of a qualified health practitioner who is familiar with intestinal cleansing and with treating Candida successfully. This practitioner should monitor their progress while cleansing, and adapt the program to meet their individual needs. **This is particularly important with Candida because it creates so many complicating factors**.

Following are important guidelines for cleansers who have an overgrowth of Candida:

- ❑ Make every attempt to pass the pH tests, knowing that many who have Candida overgrowth may be unable to do so.
- ❑ Drink vegetable broths in place of juices.
- ❑ Do not have fruit or sweet vegetable juices on the Cleanse. Use only water with the psyllium-bentonite shakes.
- ❑ Throughout all phases of cleansing, take one-fourth (1/4) teaspoon of the more acid-forming probiotic formula at least one hour before bedtime, one-half hour after each set of herbs, and one-half hour after each meal.
- ❑ On the last week of the Cleanse take the less-acid probiotic formula *along with* the above.
- ❑ After completing the Cleanse, discontinue using the more acid-forming probiotic and take four (4) serving sizes of the less acid probiotic, three (3) times daily after meals, for approximately three (3) weeks.
- ❑ Begin use of the formula for renewing or rebuilding the bowel wall approximately three (3) hours after the last psyllium shake.

Since there is generally a strong emotional component with an overgrowth of Candida, it is critical to do some honest self-evaluation while cleansing, and make a strong effort to apply the mental and emotional cleansing principles discussed in Book 2 of this series, in Chapter 9: "Optimize Your Cleanse." You may also want to secure the assistance of a trained professional who can help you uncover the subconscious emotions that are the primal cause of the overgrowth. Cleansing is a very good start, and the use of breathwork can enhance this process significantly.

Friendly Bacteria Essential

Failure to replace friendly bacteria after cleansing, or fasting, or after using strong laxatives, and especially after taking antibiotics, can cause an overgrowth of pathogenic microorganisms and long-term future health problems. Obtaining the correct bacteria is difficult, for most people have been programmed to use **acid-forming bacteria as a replacement for the less acid-forming bacteria we were given by our mothers in breast milk.** This is so critical that with the assistance of my good friend Dr. Khem M. Shahani at the University of Nebraska, I developed one of the few probiotics available that contain bacteria that are natural to humans. It is designed to use during and after cleansing. It may also be used any time you sense that your friendly bacteria may have been weakened due to improper diet, stress, or even when you have been exposed to a "bug" you don't want to catch! Even when persons have started to 'come down' with something, using this formula has been reported to speed recovery time. With today's diet and lifestyles, using the correct bacterial formula is essential for good health.

What are the correct friendly bacteria? Some persons have taken large amounts of *acidophilus*, thinking they were helping their bodies. Yet even doctors disagree about the uses of *Lactobacillus acidophilus*. In my opinion, *acidophilus* should be used as an agent to remove pathogenic bacteria, or sparingly, in combination with other bacteria that produce a higher pH. Everyone agrees that *Lactobacillus*, such as *acidophilus*, has an important role in the treatment of pathogenic bacteria such as *E. coli*, *Salmonella*, etc. However, it also produces an acid by-product with a pH between 3.0 and 4.5. Because of this extreme acidity, bowel problems are likely to occur if a more alkaline-forming formula, such as one containing *Bifidobacterium*, is not used after taking *acidophilus*.

My experience indicates that **the best *general probiotic formula* consists of *Bifidobacterium infantis*, along with a variety of other bifidobacteria, as well as a small percentage of *acidophilus*.** *Bifidobacterium infantis* is found in healthy, breast-fed infants, and is possibly the basic foundational bacteria for the human species. Since I began using this new type of bacteria, my health has moved up another notch. It is designed to replenish the normal, friendly bacteria and should be used any time your system has been weakened due to stress, poor diet, and use of antibiotics, birth control pills, or other medical treatments.

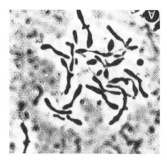

B. bifidum

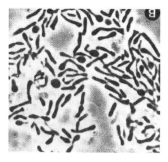

B. longum

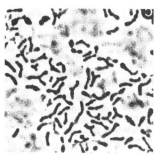

B. breve

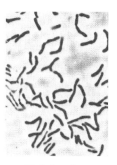

B. infantis

I have also created a *second probiotic formula* to be used when we have symptoms indicating the presence of pathogenic microorganisms. This probiotic contains potent acid-forming bacteria and must be replaced with the less acid-forming formula. Symptoms indicating a need for the acid-forming formula may include excessive gas, food poisoning, nutritional deficiencies, *Candida albicans*, bacterial infections, systemic toxicity, and a weakened immune system. The bacteria in this formula are known to stimulate the production of immunologic factors; this includes interlukin-1a, and tumor necrosis factor-1 by microphages. [101] They are also known to help eliminate various species of pathogenic bacteria, including: *Staphylococcus, Salmonella, Pseudomonas, Shigella, Klebsiella pneumoniae, Sarcina lutea, Vibrio comma (Asiatic cholera),* and *Escherichia(E.) coli.*[102,103] The second formula is specifically for yeast problems, as well as for addressing specific pathogenic bacteria such as those listed above.

How to Shrink the Abdomen, Repair Prolapsus

A thick and dangerous mucoid buildup in the intestinal tract, as seen in the famous "beer belly," causes damage to surrounding tissues.[104] Once the mucoid layers are removed, the seriously stretched intestines are still soft and flabby. But there is hope for a normal and healthy look – blessed are herbs!

After cleansing, white oak bark and ginger root, when used together, can help to draw the flesh back to its original position. Take three (3) capsules of white oak bark with three (3) capsules of ginger root three (3) times daily on an empty stomach. Those with a prolapsus should use a slant board along with these herbs after completing the Cleanse. While on the slant board, gently massage the intestines upwards. Do this two or three times daily or as needed. Follow your intuition.

The same herbs are also suggested for those with prolapsus of the transverse colon along with the use of a slant board. Lie on the slant board with the head down, and gently stroke the abdomen, especially the transverse colon, towards the head. Reach as deep as you can and draw

---

[101] N. Rangavajhyala, K. M. Shahani, G. Sridevi, and S. Srikumaran, "Nonlipopolysaccharide Component(s) of *Lactobacillus acidophilus* Stimulate(s) the Production of Interleukin-a and Tumor Necrosis Factor-q by Murine Macrophages," *Nutrition and Cancer,* Vol. 27 or 28 (2), pg. 130-134.

[102] Khem M. Shahani, Jayantkumar R. Vakil, Rarnesh Chandra Chandan, United States Patent # 3,689,640, Sept. 5, 1972.

[103] K. M. Shahani, J. R. Vakil, and A. Kilara, *Natural Antibotic Activity of Lactobacillus acidophilus and bulgaricus.* Information on this research available from the Department of Food Sciences and Technology, University of Nebraska, Lincoln, Nebraska 68583.

[104] This stretching may cause a "Leaky Bowel Syndrome," which is discussed in Book 2 in Chapter 6: "Impaired Digestion and Its Outcomes."

your intestinal tubes upwards. Visualize them staying in place. Remember, your mind is the controlling factor in your life. Once your subconscious mind accepts your suggestion as true, it will become a reality.

Potential Problems with Cleansing

Approximately 1 out of 5,000 people who complete a full Cleanse have some difficulty after the Cleanse. This may include feelings of fullness, as though something is trapped in the gut, constipation, or other various digestive or other disturbances. Symptoms are multifarious and unique. One person, for example, was extremely upset because he was left with a swollen lymph gland near the groin; it took several weeks for it to dissipate. Some of these people have temporarily lost sight of all the wonderful benefits they obtained, and made the mistake of focusing only on their immediate and temporary crisis with fear and anger. For anyone who experiences something along these lines, it is important to keep the big picture in mind.

Generally what is going on here is that while on the Cleanse, these people entered a very deep cleansing cycle, but they stopped their cleansing prior to its natural completion. Therefore, toxic debris, that was still in circulation and destined to be eliminated, was trapped – it could not escape. When this occurs, the body is forced to remove the debris the hard way – by breaking the particles down into molecular acids and gradually removing them via whatever channel is available.

The very best action would have been to go back into cleansing and allow the body to complete what it was trying to do – dump the garbage. However, partly due to the fear that our society and conventional medicine instills about fasting, some people have jumped to the conclusion that something was wrong with the Cleanse. Some – very few, fortunately – go to the nearest medical doctors for help. This has proven to be the worst mistake they can make, for medical doctors know as much about fasting, herbs, nutrition, and healing crises as *you* know about the ancient civilization that disappeared from Mars, maybe even less. And for these people, when they follow advice from those who are uninformed or misinformed it always takes longer, sometimes much longer, to overcome their present crisis.

Knowing that approximately one out of six children[105] (not even including adults) in America suffer from some degree from lead poisoning,

---

[105] See the Web Site "The Arc's Q & A on Lead Poisoning." (http://www.thearc.org/faqs/leadqa.html).

I have long been concerned that cleansing may uncover lead deposits. If this did occur, it could cause serious problems. Fortunately, even out of all the many tens of thousands who have used intestinal and colon cleanses, not a single case has been reported to me. But it can and does happen to those who water fast. I know, for it happened to me.

Heavy Metals

Heavy metals can gradually accumulate in the body over a period of years; the body has some capacity to store them without any obvious incident. But if pockets of heavy metals are exposed by whatever means, they can cause severe reactions and actually damage cells and organs. Many people have heavy metals stored in their kidneys, bones, and mucus. If an individual uncovers a pocket of stored heavy metals, the symptoms are severe and possibly dangerous. If anyone suspects he or she is experiencing symptoms due to heavy metals toxicity, I would strongly suggest immediately contacting my office for information on an effective and relatively inexpensive program for detoxifying from heavy metals.

I doubt if medical doctors would know what to do if someone who had been water fasting, developed symptoms of lead poisoning, and tried to explain their symptoms to Mr. M.D. I was one of those persons who uncovered heavy metal – lead – while water fasting, and I was devastated. It took me more than a year to realize what the problem was and then, out of desperation, I spent months doing research and finally developed a program that worked remarkably well to cleanse the body of heavy metals toxicity.

Will that experience prevent me from water fasting? Absolutely not. In fact, while I am writing this, I am on another water fast. But the experience revealed to me that I need to go deeper than what I had ever imagined before. Heavy metals are dangerous, and wherever they settle in the body, there is a time bomb ready to go off. I believe that many dis-eases in our society are the result of heavy metals poisoning, and this includes many cancer scenarios. I also believe that many people die from heavy metals. The worst of all is lead, and this information has been deliberately covered up. If you see an elderly person who gradually loses weight and then suddenly falls apart and dies within a few days or weeks, I would certainly consider that his or her stored heavy metals had been uncovered, with lethal results.

As for myself, I want all heavy metals out of my body, as well as everything else that could cause a weakness in my mind or body. And I will use water and juice fasting along with my heavy-metal detox to remove them. I am, however, being very careful about this.

Read below, and if you have at least the first three symptoms listed, then you may be suffering from *heavy metals poisoning*. If so, call immediately if you want to know about my **heavy-metal detox program**.

A Few Signs of Heavy Metals Toxicity[106]

♦ Extreme and unusual weakness
♦ Fear that something is dreadfully wrong
♦ Sudden and unusual mental incoherence
♦ Sudden lymphatic congestion or blockage
♦ Sudden and unusual pain in kidneys
♦ Sudden and unusual pain in liver
♦ Sudden and unusual edema
♦ Sudden, unusual, and extreme incoordination
♦ Sudden and unusual heart palpitations (severe)
♦ Unusual headaches
♦ Unusual bone pain
♦ Unquenchable thirst
♦ Numbness, coldness, and poor circulation in extremities.

---

[106] As noted on page 20, the "diamond bullets" indicate warning points.

CHAPTER 11

DIRECTIONS FOR THE MOST EFFECTIVE INTESTINAL CLEANSING PROGRAM

"A good reliable set of bowels is worth more to a man than any quantity of brains."

– Henry Wheeler Shaw

The success of my full intestinal and total body Cleanse Program has been so astounding that we have come to believe that its success cannot be totally attributed to just the removal of mucoid plaque and toxicants. Over the years we have seen overwhelming evidence that the Cleanse also "pulls out" negative consciousness, which has become stuck in physical tissue. I have researched this phenomenon for many years and my conclusions have been supported by thousands of testimonies, which reveal major changes in attitudes and emotions. People simply released old negative thought patterns while cleansing, which undoubtedly had attributed to their past dis-ease conditions. It is important to keep this in mind and **encourage emotions to surface; just do so with the expectation that when emotions surface, the experience will be temporary and highly beneficial.**

Important Points[107]

❑ **Do pH Tests!** Most people in the Western World are deficient in electrolytes. This is one of the main factors contributing towards dis-ease. If one is deficient in electrolytes while cleansing or fasting, then the cleansing process will be sluggish and inefficient. It may also contribute towards the weakening of the liver, kidneys,

---

[107] As noted on page 20, the "box bullets" indicate informational points, or instructions.

and other organs. No one should chance it: Make certain that you have full electrolyte reserves before cleansing. Please follow the simple directions for testing your pH.

❑ **Do a three-week Cleanse using the Gentle (or Mildest and Gentle) Phase** before continuing to the Power or Master Phase. Preparation for the Master Phase of the Cleanse is critical for optimal success. This vital first period helps eliminate an incredible amount of toxins gradually and safely without placing too much stress upon your vital organs.

❑ **Listen to your body!** Every person reacts differently to every herb, food, program, etc. The only one that knows for sure what it needs is your own, special body, so listen to it carefully. **Do not cleanse until you feel that it is right for you. Your body is your responsibility and no one else's.**

❑ **Always stand up slooowly!** The deeper you go into cleansing, the greater the amounts of toxins, excess proteins and mucus that enter the bloodstream, and the more sluggish circulation can become. Thus it may take longer for oxygen to reach the brain when you stand up. Always sit up first, take several deep breaths, and then slowly stand. Some people have become dizzy; some have actually passed out. Do not let this happen to you.

❑ **No salt!** Never use any kind of inorganic salt, either orally or rectally, when doing the Cleanse. Absolutely nothing is more harmful to the cleansing process. Large amounts of salt can calcify the mucoid plaque and injure the intestinal mucosa. Nothing will stop cleansing more abruptly than salt. If you're a heavy salt consumer, cleansing will be slower and the elimination of mucoid plaque will be minimal.

❑ **Do not allow yourself to feel bad.** Assist your body's elimination processes as needed, with colonics, or enemas. Herbs for specific organ support, fresh raw organic juices, or chiropractic, massage, acupuncture or breathwork sessions may also be used as desired. If cleansing reactions persist, you may need to go back to an easier phase of the Cleanse. See Chapter 10, under "Four Phases of Cleansing Adaptable to Individual Needs."

❑ **Bacteria -** Over the years, we have found that it is *essential* to take a probiotic during all phases of the Program except the Mildest Phase. For some, whose bodies are very depeleted, it may be important to take friendly bacteria during the Mildest Phase also. Many choose to take it on the Mildest Phase as on the other phases, just to be certain they have adequate friendly bacteria in their systems. Continuous intake of this probiotic helps prevent yeasts and other pathogens from obtaining a foothold. It also helps prevent constipation and hunger after the Cleanse. Take one capsule a half an hour before bedtime. Do not use *Lactobacillus* products, such as *acidophilus*, for they produce too much acid, and contribute to an electrolyte deficiency.

Notes for the Hypersensitive or Universal Reactor

Be sure to read the check-off list under "Important Points" at the beginning of this Chapter, and do the pH tests. For those who are extremely sensitive to foods, herbs, and practically everything else, who are "Universal Reactors," are very weak, very ill, very old, or are just plain nervous about cleansing, it would be good to do a few tests before beginning. For example:

❑ Try only half (1/2) of a capsule. Wait a few hours and see how you feel. The next time take a whole capsule. Gradually increase.

❑ When you make your first shake, try it with only a half (1/2) teaspoon of psyllium (or less) and no bentonite. Gradually increase. With later shakes, try adding a small portion of bentonite.

Following these gradual methods of using the herbs and other elements of the Cleanse will help you avoid any problems, and help condition the body to handle larger doses. Increase at your own speed. All of the herbs are very natural, gentle, and safe, but you'll have more confidence if you increase slowly. You can also alternate between the Mildest and Gentle Phases, listening to your body's needs.

Note: If you have a serious health condition, consult your naturopathic doctor, or another health expert before cleansing. You may also check my Web Site for further cleanse information (http://www.cleanse.net).

Items Needed for the Cleanse

The Herbal formulas
Extra-thick bentonite
General-use probiotic

Psyllium*
Shaker jar
pH papers

*Note: I recommend a psyllium that has been flash-heat sterilized, in contrast to most on the market today, which are ETO (ethylene tri-oxide), or EO (ethylene oxide) treated. There is evidence that EO and ETO residues may be associated with nausea, headaches, neurological damage and cancer development.[108] Psyllium that has not been adequately sterilized is also very likely to present a serious health risk, due to the many contaminants routinely found in the raw product, most of which comes from India.

Step 1 – Complete the pH Test, Build the Alkaline Reserve

How to Test Your pH

This three-part pH test helps indicate an electrolyte deficiency, which could inhibit the cleansing process and initiate unnecessary or even harmful cleansing reactions. If you do not pass the pH test, you can still do the Mildest Phase or the Gentle Phase. However, it is essential that you have a full alkaline electrolyte reserve before doing the Power Phase or the Master Phase. You will need pH papers, pen/pencil, paper, and 1 lemon. The tests must be done at least two (2) hours after meals.

Part #1 – The Saliva Test

Thoroughly wet the end of a small strip of pH paper with your saliva and compare its color to the nearest color indicated on the pH paper dispenser. The color chart may not always match the readings exactly, just use your best judgment. Record the date and the results on a piece of paper.

Interpreting Part #1

6.0 or below - Indicates a seriously depleted electrolyte condition and potential problems while exercising, cleaning, or fasting. You must replenish your alkaline reserve before doing any cleansing, fasting or strenuous exercise. DO NOT EXERCISE STRENUOUSLY! Perform Part #2.

---

[108] From research conducted by the Seveso II Council Directive, See the Web Site: (http://mahbsrv.jrc.it/Framework-Seveso2-Annex1.html). Refer to page 17 of 37 under Ethylene oxide: "Neurological disorders and even death after exposure have been reported. Probable human carcinogen."

6.1 - 6.3 - Indicates depletion. May not be serious, but electrolytes are low. Perform Part #2.

6.4 - 6.8 - Passed Part # 1. This is a very good sign. Perform Part #2.

6.9 or higher - Something may have interfered with the reading, such as stress or excitement. Wait about one hour and test again. If the results remain the same, it indicates psychological stress that is so deep that it is causing metabolic stress. It could also be related to old drugs, emotions, infections, parasites, etc. Perform Part #2.

Part #2 – The Lemon Test

This test can be done immediately after the saliva test. Squeeze the juice of one half (1/2)of a lemon into two (2) ounces of water and drink without sweeteners. Swish the juice in the mouth once just before swallowing. Wait for 60 seconds, and then begin a series of six (6) saliva readings with the pH papers. Record each reading. At least one of the last three readings must show a passing result to pass this part of the test

Interpreting Part #2

8 or higher - You passed. This indicates that the liver has stored adequate electrolytes to buffer the acids in the mouth. This is a positive health indicator. If, during Part #1 of the test, the saliva reading was between 6.4 and 6.8, and you passed the lemon test, then it is safe to cleanse or fast. Proceed to Part #3.

7.5 - 8.0 - You barely passed and you may cleanse, but your electrolyte reserve is not fully charged. You should strive to increase your reserve during the Mildest and Gentle Phases.

7.0 - 7.4 - Indicates that you have some reserve of alkaline minerals, but not as much as needed. Work diligently on increasing your electrolyte reserve during the Mildest and Gentle Phases. Do not go into deeper phases until you have a reading above 7.5.

6.9 or below, but higher than the reading in Part 1 - Indicates that there is some reserve, but it is minimal. This indicates that you are moving towards a chronic, dis-eased condition. Use only the Mildest Phase until you pass the pH test. Proceed to Part #3. Support from an expert health practitioner is advised!

143

Part #3 – The Urine Test

To complete this test you'll need to devote a day to eating only vegetables and their juices (100% alkaline-forming foods). Have no grains, dairy, meat, coffee, or fruits; and do not exercise strenuously. The next morning, wet the pH paper in a mid-stream of urine. Record your result.

Interpreting Part #3

7.0 or above - You passed. It means that your body has so much extra electrolyte reserve that it is eliminating the excess through the urine.

6.5 - 6.9 - Indicates some depletion, although it is not yet too serious. The body is storing some electrolytes but is releasing some as well. Work on increasing your electrolytes during the Mildest and Gentle Phases. As long as you passed the first two parts of the test, it is safe to cleanse deeply.

5.6 - 6.4 - Depletion is more serious. Acid accumulation is greater than your alkaline reserve. This means that your body may be killing its own cells to retrieve the electrolytes it needs to keep your body alive. It is a sign that you are moving towards a dis-ease. Focus on replenishing your electrolyte storehouse before cleansing. Then, be sure to pass all parts of the pH test. Caution is advised while cleansing.

5.6 or below - A pH in this range indicates the body is very depleted and has no storage of electrolytes. It is unlikely that you would have passed Part #1 and Part #2. Do not attempt any cleansing or fasting beyond the Mildest Phase. Some type of chronic or degenerative dis-ease has probably already developed.

Those who did not pass the pH test should stop eating acid food, and eat mostly vegetables, particularly those that are high in *organic electrolytes:* sodium, potassium, calcium, and magnesium. Drink plenty of fresh organic juices. Use organic electrolyte supplements. Cleanse using the Mildest Phase only until you pass all three parts of the test. You can begin the Gentle Phase once you have built up your alkaline reserves and passed the entire pH test. Then you can continue with the deeper cleansing of the Power or Master Phases.

Note: Urine tests during cleansing - After you begin the Power or Master Phase, and for a few people, the Gentle Phase, the body will be removing stored acids. The deeper the cleansing, the more acid the urine becomes. Checking your urine pH during these phases will not indicate your true electrolyte status. In other words, it's useless. However, Part #2 (the lemon test) should continue to be accurate.

Summary of pH Test Results

Indicators of serious mineral depletion & poor health	Signs of good health & full reserve of electrolytes
Saliva pH between meals is below 6.1.	Saliva pH between meals is above 6.4 to 6.8.
Lemon test is below 7.0 pH.	Lemon test reveals 8.0 or above.
After eating 100% alkaline-forming foods in a 24-hour period, the next morning's urine pH is below 7.0.	After eating 100% alkaline-forming foods in a 24-hour period the next morning's urine pH is 7.0 or above.
After eating 100% acid-forming foods, the next morning's urine pH is above 7.0.	After eating 100% acid-forming foods, the next morning's urine pH is 6.0 or below.
Smell of ammonia in urine.	

Note: For more details about pH, refer to *Cleanse & Purify,* Book 2.

Rebuilding the Alkaline Reserve

❑ Eliminate all acid-forming foods.
❑ Consume only alkaline-forming foods.
❑ Eat only food that is organically grown; remember, commercially-grown foods are deficient in minerals and other nutrients.
❑ Drink about 16 ounces of fresh vegetable juice three or more times daily, especially carrot, celery, beet, and kale.
❑ Take organic electrolyte supplements containing dehydrated beet juice, celery, carrot, and kale and goat whey.
❑ Drinking vegetable broth is very good for building electrolyte levels. Instructions to make this may be found at the end of Appendix 1.

Proper diet is one of the most important resources for rebuilding the alkaline reserve. For a list of acid- and alkaline-forming foods, see Appendix 1 in the back of this book.

Note: Grains, legumes, and cooked roots such as potatoes will slow down the cleansing process. Dairy products and meat destroy the cleansing process.

Step 2 – Preparing to Start the Cleanse

Familiarize yourself with the instructions under Step 3 for all four cleanse phases. Based on your pH test results, decide whether you will start with the Mildest or the Gentle Phase.

The Day Before Starting the Cleanse

Your last regular meal should be lunch. The evening meal should consist of fresh, raw fruit. This is a good habit to get into: making your dinner of fresh fruit only; you will find that you sleep better at night, and your body will cleanse itself while you sleep. There are some who feel that you could put a stop to one-half your ailments by doing that alone!

Note: You may also wish to refer to Chapter 9 to remind yourself about the details of the different Phases.

Determining the Amounts of Herbs to Take

The proper amounts of the herbs for *you* must be determined by you; **according to how *your* body responds.** The average person takes one serving size of each formula. The goal is to have three to five (3-5) stools per day on all phases and they should be soft, yet formed. If you take an enema in the morning and evening, then you may need no other bowel elimination.

- ❑ If your stools are sticky, hard, or dry, or you experience constipation, increase your dose of the herbs slowly until stools are soft, yet formed.
- ❑ If your stools are loose or runny, cut down on the amount of herbs you are taking. If your stools are loose or runny with less than one serving size of each formula, you need to take a special herbal formula.
- ❑ A highly constipated person may safely take 17 servings or more of each formula per day. Dosage should be increased slowly, noting how the body responds.

How to Make and Use a Psyllium-Bentonite Shake

To the 16-ounce shaker bottle add:

- ❑ 1 Tablespoon **Extra Thick** Liquid Bentonite (or more),
- ❑ 1-2 **tea**spoons Psyllium Husk Powder (Note: This is a <u>tea</u>spoon, *not* a tablespoon.),
- ❑ 8 to 12 ounces of water (preferably distilled).

Then place the lid on the jar and shake vigorously.

- ❑ Drink immediately, as the shake will begin to thicken.
- ❑ Drink 8 ounces of water after the shake.

Note: If you do not use extra-thick bentonite, about six (6) tablespoons of an average hydrated bentonite are needed.

Note: Two to four (2-4) ounces of the water may be substituted with fruit juice. Those who have sugar or yeast problems must not have fruit juices.

When to Take Supplements

Most supplements should be taken 15 minutes prior to taking the herbs or just before a meal. In this way the body can utilize their maximum nutritional value. See "The Options," in Chapter 9: "The Powerful Ingredients of a Superb Intestinal Cleanse."

Step 3 – Cleansing

What to Eat While Cleansing

While on any of the phases, eat no meat, dairy products, salt, sugar, or foods with added sugar in them. Get into the habit of reading labels; this will help you know what you're actually consuming. Have no fried food or foods cooked in oils. Limit your oil intake to cold-pressed organic olive oil or flax seed oil. Honey, organic maple syrup, stevia, and date sugar sweeteners are acceptable. Eat as many raw foods as your body desires. Eat all the fruit, salads, and raw or cooked vegetables you want. Those with a sugar or yeast problem should eat only vegetables. Try to have at least one raw meal per day and plenty of fresh vegetable juice and/or fruit juice. Drink water as often as you like except during meals. Fresh-made vegetable mineral broth is a fantastic food resource to help provide electrolyte minerals while cleansing, and may be taken regularly.

If you feel that you need to eat something heavy, have the following but limit them to only once or twice a week: grains, beans, potatoes, or squash. Soak all grains and beans overnight before you lightly cook them. Millet and quinoa, though more alkaline-forming grains, should also be limited to once or twice a week. Remember, **root vegetables, grains, and legumes slow down the cleansing.**

Carrot juice is a wonderful, nutrient-rich food, but it is fairly high in natural sugar. Therefore, those who need to restrict their sugar intake may need to dilute it with water or other vegetable juices. Fruit juices may also need to be diluted. You can eliminate fruit juice entirely if you choose. Fresh, non-sweet green juices may be used freely.

Fresh, raw fruits and vegetables may be used as snacks. Take snacks 45 minutes after a shake or 30 minutes after herbs.

If you follow these suggestions, you'll condition your body for cleansing in a gradual way, which may keep you from feeling down, sluggish, or toxic.

The Protein Myth

Far more people are sick because of too much protein rather than not enough. Protein is in all fruits and vegetables. Though meat eaters consume more protein, they actually have more protein deficiencies than vegetarians because of dysfunctional liver and digestion resulting from their intake of too many acid-forming foods. Yet there are some who may need a little more protein. I recommend that these people take an ultimate food chlorophyll supplement.

Note: Studies have shown that organically grown produce has as much as 300% more nutrition than commercially grown produce. Health cannot be maintained without an adequate supply of minerals.

Common Facts for All Phases of Cleansing

- ❑ Always begin the day with a psyllium-bentonite shake.
- ❑ One and one-half (1-1/2) hours later, take the herbs.
- ❑ One and one-half (1-1/2) hours later, take another shake, and One and one-half (1-1/2) hours after that, take herbs again.
- ❑ Take the herbs two (2) hours after your lunch and dinner.
- ❑ On all Phases it is important that you avoid acid-forming foods.
- ❑ Drink all the fresh, organic juice you wish, especially carrot and celery juice, and fresh greens.
- ❑ Consider using organic electrolyte supplements, ultimate food chlorophyll formulas, or trace minerals supplements.

> **Note**: Always use **organically grown** vegetables and fruits.

> Note: Never take herbs with the psyllium shake. Each will significantly counteract the other.

> **Note: It is essential to *follow the directions*, for *each* Phase.**

Mildest Phase

On this phase you will concentrate on rebuilding your alkaline reserves.

Mildest Phase Facts

- ❑ Two and one-half (2-1/2) alkaline-forming meals daily. The half meal should include fresh fruit only.
- ❑ Two (2) psyllium-bentonite shakes. Begin your day with a shake.
- ❑ Three (3) sets of herbs. The average dosage is one serving size of each formula or more according to your need. Take each set of herbs one and one-half hours (1-1/2) after each shake and two (2) hours after each meal.
- ❑ One (1) or more servings of the more alkaline-producing probiotic. Take this one-half (1/2) hour before bed.

Mildest Phase Example	
6:00 A.M.Psyllium Shake	3:00 P.M. Psyllium Shake
7:30 A.M. Breakfast	4:30 P.M. Dinner*
10:30 A.M. Herbs	7:00 P.M. Herbs
12:00 P.M. Lunch*	8:30 P.M. Probiotic
1:30 P.M. Herbs	

Gentle Phase

This is a very important phase. **No one should begin the more powerful phases without first doing the Gentle Phase** (or a combination of the Mildest and Gentle Phases) **for three (3) weeks.** And each subsequent time you cleanse, you should begin with at least a week of this phase. Removing too much waste too rapidly places a heavy and unnecessary burden on your organs. What took months, years, or a lifetime to create cannot be cleaned up in a few weeks. It usually requires about a week for the herbs to prepare the mucoid plaque to be removed, and during this time, you can also release a large amount of toxic waste, thereby reducing potential difficulties when you do the deeper phases.

Gentle Phase Facts

❑ Two (2) highly alkaline-forming meals daily, such as fruits and vegetables, salad greens.

❑ Three (3) psyllium-bentonite shakes. Begin the day with a shake.

❑ Five (5) sets of herbs daily. Take each set of herbs one-and-a-half hours (1-1/2) after each shake and two (2) hours after each meal.

❑ One (1) or more of the alkaline-producing probiotic. Take one-half (½) hour before bed and five (5) minutes after each meal. (See "Gentle Phase Example"chart, which follows).

❑ All the juice you wish.

❑ If you have cleansing reactions, take enemas. Enemas will also speed up the cleansing process.

❑ After using the Gentle Phase for three (3) weeks, proceed to either the Power or Master Phase.

Note: Truly healthy people do not have mucoid plaque.

Note: Limit citrus juice. For some people, citrus, especially orange juice, is hard on the kidneys. Orange juice may also affect their calcium balance.

Gentle Phase Example	
6:00 A.M.Psyllium Shake	2:00 P.M. Herbs
7:30 A.M. Herbs	3:30 P.M. Psyllium Shake
9:00 A.M. Psyllium Shake	5:00 P.M. Herbs
10:30 A.M. Herbs	6:30 P.M. Dinner*
12:00 P.M. Lunch*	8:30 P.M. Probiotic

*For many whose bodies are very depleted and toxic, it is an excellent idea to take additional servings of the probiotic, five (5) minutes after each meal.

Power Phase

The Power Phase is exactly like the Gentle Phase except that one of the meals is replaced with a psyllium shake. Having four shakes and less food will speed up the cleansing. However, it is not nearly as powerful as the Master Phase, although it is a very powerful phase. You may remove a significant buildup of toxins, pathogens, and perhaps many feet of mucoid plaque.

Take an enema two to three (2-3) hours before going to bed, and whenever a cleansing reaction arises. Enemas are not an absolute requirement, but are very highly recommended during both the Power and Master Phases and will speed up the cleansing process and make your cleanse most effective. (Refer to Chapter 13: "How to Take an Enema" if this is foreign territory for you. Don't knock enemas until you've read the chapter and tried one!)

People Should Not Do the Power Phase Until They Have the Following

- ❑ A good alkaline reserve (they should pass all the pH tests),
- ❑ No cleanse reactions during the final three (3) days of the Gentle Phase,
- ❑ A strong conviction the time is right to switch to this phase.

Remember, your health is *your* responsibility!

Power Phase Facts

- ❑ One (1) highly alkaline-forming meal.
- ❑ Four (4) psyllium-bentonite shakes.

151

- Five (5) sets of herbs. Dosage is the same as on other phases.
- Take two (2) or more of the alkaline-producing probiotic, one-half (½) hour before bed and five (5) minutes after the meal.
- All the juice you wish − carrot/celery/kale juice are especially healthful.
- At least 1 enema daily is recommended. If you have cleansing reactions, take enemas. Enemas will also speed up the cleansing process.

> Note: If you're having a cleansing reaction (discomfort, diarrhea, vomiting, headaches, fatigue, or dizziness), don't move to a higher phase. In fact, you may choose to move to a milder phase. See Chapter 12: "Cleansing Reactions."

Power Phase Example	
Enema	1:30 P.M. Herbs
6:00 A.M. Psyllium Shake	3:00 P.M. Psyllium Shake
7:30 A.M. Herbs	4:30 P.M. Herbs
9:00 A.M. Psyllium Shake	6:00 P.M. Dinner*
10:30 A.M. Herbs	8:00 P.M. Herbs
12:00 P.M. Psyllium Shake	9:00 P.M. Probiotic

*For many whose bodies are very depleted and toxic, it is an excellent idea to take additional servings of the probiotic, five (5) minutes after each meal.

The Master Phase- Let's Go for It (No Meals)

The Master Phase is the ultimate Cleansing Phase. This is where people receive their most transforming benefits. The Power Phase is a good test to see if they are ready for the Master Phase. Most experienced Cleansers can skip the Power Phase, for they know how their bodies will respond.

People Should Not Do the Master Phase Until They Have the Following

- A good alkaline reserve (they should pass all the pH tests prior to the Gentle Phase).
- No cleansing reactions for the last three (3) days of the Power Phase.

❏ An intuitive feeling that doing this phase is the right thing to do. Remember, your health is *your* responsibility! Use your "inner knowing."

Note: Before doing the Master Phase, it is a good idea to do the Power Phase for two or three days to test your body. If you have cleansing reactions while on the Power Phase, then you may not be ready to do the Master Phase. When you can do the Power Phase for two days without having a cleansing reaction, then you are ready to do the Master Phase.

Note: If you feel weak and tired on any of the Cleanse Phases, it may be because you are either too toxic or depleted of electrolytes, not because you're not eating enough. First, drink about 1 quart of water within 30 minutes. If the problem persists, then take an enema. If this doesn't work, then take a coffee enema. If that doesn't work, review the material on Cleansing Reactions in Chapter 12. If the coffee enema makes you feel better, it wasn't the caffeine, it was because the liver was toxic and the enema cleared the liver. This indicates that the liver needs help. Read "The Liver, Cleansing and Rejuvenating the Vital Organ."

Note: **Diabetics, hypoglycemics, or those with yeast or sugar problems** should not use fruit juices or even carrot juice while cleansing. They should drink vegetable broths.

Master Phase Facts

❏ Eat no foods during this time, but drink all the fresh vegetable juice you want, especially carrot/celery/kale juice.
❏ Five (5) psyllium-bentonite shakes daily.
❏ Five (5) sets of herbs daily. Dosage – same as on other phases.
❏ Take two (2) or more of the alkaline-producing probiotic, one-half (½) hour before bed.
❏ Drink all the juice you wish.
❏ Two (2) enemas daily are recommended.
❏ While Cleansing, if your energy is low, you can take ultimate food chlorophyll formulas or trace minerals supplements. (See "The Options" at the end of Chapter 9: The Powerful Ingredients of a Superb Intestinal Cleanse)

Note: For those who refuse to take enemas, you may need to increase the amount of the herbs to assure *at least three (3)* bowel movements per day.

Master Phase Example	
6:00 A.M. Psyllium Shake	1:30 P.M. Herbs
6:15 A.M. Enema	3:00 P.M. Psyllium Shake
7:30 A.M. Herbs	4:30 P.M. Herbs
9:00 A.M. Psyllium Shake	6:00 P.M. Psyllium Shake
10:30 A.M. Herbs	6:30 P.M. Enema
12:00 P.M. Psyllium Shake	7:30 P.M. Herbs
	9:00 P.M. Probiotic

Step 4 – Ending the Cleanse

If you did only the Gentle or Mild Phase, just increase the more alkaline-producing probiotic and eat well. Those who used the Power or Master Phase should do the following:

> **Note:** The most important thing you can do after cleansing and fasting is to: 1) **Drink extra water.** It is common for people to become dehydrated after they begin to eat again. It is far better to drink too much water than not enough. 2) Avoid constipation. The essentials for healthy bowels that move adequately include: enough water, bacteria, and fiber. If necessary, take an enema or herbs.

7th Day

1. After 3 P.M., stop taking the shakes. In their place, drink fresh vegetable juice or eat fresh fruit – apples are ideal, for they assist the bowels to move.
2. In the evening, either drink fresh juice for supper, eat all the fruit you want, *or* make a vegetable broth.
3. Vegetable broth. Sip slowly. Do not mix fruits and vegetables.
4. Two (2) hours after "supper," take the normal amount of herbs.
5. Take 4 of the more alkaline-producing probiotic.

8th Day

1. In the morning, drink between 24 and 32 ounces of water, and then take 1 shake *without* bentonite.
2. You should have a bowel movement in the morning. If you do not, take an enema.
3. Have breakfast. Any fresh fruit would be fine, but do not mix citrus or melons with any other fruits. Avoid cooked food and

dairy products. After eating, take four (4) servings of my more alkaline-forming probiotic formula.

4. Lunch should consist of fresh fruit, lightly steamed vegetables, or freshly made soup. After eating, take four (4) servings of my more alkaline-forming probiotic formula.

5. Supper should consist of fresh raw salad. After eating, take four (4) servings of my more alkaline-forming probiotic formula.

6. Two hours after supper, take the herbs. You may also reduce your normal dosage if that seems appropriate to you. For at least five (5) days following the eighth day, take two to three (2-3) of the more alkaline-producing probiotic after lunch and dinner.

Note: One cannot maintain good health unless one has at least two (2) bowel movements daily. Ideally, a person should have a BM first thing in the morning and within 30 minutes after a meal. Constipation is one of the primary promoters of *poor* health.

9th Day and After

1. Maintain a diet of raw and lightly steamed vegetables and all the fruit you desire. Heavy intake of apples is recommended during this period. Have one cleanse shake each morning (without bentonite), followed with herbs one and one-half (1-½) hours later, for at least seven (7) or more days following Cleanse completion.

2. Then maintain a transition diet of 80% alkaline-forming and 20% acid-forming foods, and 60% to 80% raw foods. Gradually cut out the herbs.

3. Congratulations! May good health always be yours!

About Constipation

In America, constipation is epidemic. It is essential to our health to keep our bowels moving. Some people will find that after the Cleanse they have no more problems. Others need more help. There have been thousands of people who have used the same herbs we use for the Cleanse to keep their bowels moving. After a period of use, many have found that they no longer needed the herbs, for their bowels had been strengthened.

However, these herbs are designed to remove the mucoid plaque; they are not designed to work as a laxative. People who need a laxative and are not using these herbs to eliminate the mucoid plaque, should try adding extra fiber and plenty of water to their diets. People are surprised to find how well their digestive system will work by drinking one very large glass of water first thing in the morning. If that doesn't do the job, then they should try one psyllium shake without bentonite in the morning after they drink their water. They should also take increased amounts of the more alkaline-forming probiotic. If they still need help, then they should continue using the herbs used during the Cleanse. Stay away from processed foods, and remember that wheat and dairy products have a detrimental effect upon the bowels, and thus upon elimination.

For optimum elimination, try to eat only two meals a day, and snack on fruit. Pineapple or apples are the only fruits I would eat after regular meals. They are beneficial digestive aids! For additional information, see Chapter 11, under "What to Eat While Cleansing," and Chapter 14: "Secrets of Good Health."

Note: If you take the same herbs for long periods, it is best to take occasional breaks. This prevents the body from becoming immune to the herbs. I would suggest that with any herbs, you take them in cycles of six (6) days and weeks, and give your body a rest from the herbs on the seventh (7th) day of each week and seventh (7th) week of a longer program. This will assure continued maximum benefits.

CHAPTER 12

CLEANSING REACTIONS

*"Since antiquity, the wisest and most successful doctors and healers, including Hippocrates himself, knew without doubt that the healing crisis marked **an essential step upon the road to recovery of vibrant health**. Passing through the healing crisis, and its less intense counterpart – the cleansing reaction – is an indicator that a significantly improved stage of health is being achieved."*

– Rich Anderson, N.D., N.M.D.

Cleansing Reaction

A cleansing reaction IS NOT the same as either a dis-ease crisis or a healing crisis. A cleansing reaction is merely a noticeable reaction triggered by too many toxins being released into the bloodstream. It could cause a temporary headache, dizziness, nausea, brain fog, weakness, lack of energy, discharges, sneezing, skin eruption, ringing in the ears, coughing or pain, flickering in the eyes, or a reappearance of other past symptoms.

Depending on the degree of toxicity in the body, there may be various cleansing reactions. These cleansing reactions differ from person to person. If people do an effective cleanse properly, they minimize cleansing reactions and never need to feel ill. Some, however, don't follow the directions; they go right into the deep phases without adequate preparation. Some people even avoid the pH tests and fail to build their electrolyte reserves. And many of these people regret their negligence. **The weaker or more toxic a person is, or the more foul the intestinal tract or sluggish the liver the greater the likelihood there will be cleansing reactions; and the more these reactions are experienced, the more the body is crying out to be cleansed.**[109]

---

[109] Ironically, the worse off people are, the less likely they are to cleanse, fast, or even change their diet. Not only do these type of people have less energy available for making *any* changes in their lives, but they also demonstrate weak wills and lower intelligence; these characteristics may likely contribute to their physical troubles. Most of the people who cleanse are highly intelligent and express a significant degree of

For most people, **the most serious cleansing reactions occur when they stand up after lying or sitting down**. When toxins are being released from our bodies, some of them enter the bloodstream in the form of excess mucus and proteins. This can cause a temporary thickening of the blood. This is normal and is necessary for the toxins to work their way out. However, this condition can slow the circulation to the point that standing up too fast can cause a pause in the flow of oxygen reaching the brain. I know two cases where people even passed out after trying to stand up. Though this does not occur too often, people should be aware that this could happen. If you find this is beginning to happen, then **make yourself stand up slowly. Keep your head down, and be careful.** This used to happen to me, but I quickly learned to stand up slowly and take deep breaths. When I was in a hurry, I walked bent over for a few seconds, until I felt normal. After several cleanses, this symptom stopped and never recurred.

People with Candidiasis are more prone to feel weak or tired while cleansing. I sincerely hope they will not let that stop them. I had Candidiasis, and on my first 9 or 10 cleanses, I didn't feel too well - not all that bad, but weak. In those early days I did not have the good sense to do bacterial implants, nor to avoid carrot and beet juice, nor even fruit juices. That was a serious mistake, and at times the Candidiasis became worse after the Cleanse. In most cases, this problem can be easily avoided if one takes large amounts of bacteria during the Cleanse.[110] By the time I developed our cleanse program, I knew what to avoid, and I knew how critical it is to reestablish the proper bacteria in the gut. After that, I experienced almost no cleansing reactions; I even felt better on the Cleanse than while eating. Not only that, but the Candidiasis symptoms gradually disappeared until they were all gone. Now I recommend that people with Candidiasis take bacteria three or four times a day during the Cleanse, and after cleansing, take it three times daily, in double dosages. They must avoid all sweet fruit and vegetable juices, and should consult with a practitioner familiar with their condition, and with digestive cleansing.

During the first few cleanses, it is not uncommon to **feel stuffed or bloated**. As the herbs soften the mucoid plaque, it swells slightly and we feel bloated. We can also feel stuffed because we have so much psyllium in

---

spiritual awareness.

[110] Bacteria in the gut help keep Candida and other yeast in check. Reduction of friendly bacteria via antibiotics or cleansing reduces competition for yeast. An effective cleanse will remove bacteria and yeast; however, it will remove bacteria first, and yeast symptoms could accelerate. Therefore, it is important that anyone who has any kind of yeast infection take extra bacteria during and after cleansing.

158

us. The bloating diminishes more and more as the mucoid plaque is eliminated. I never feel bloated anymore, no matter how much psyllium I take, but I can feel full.

Healing Crisis

The healing crisis is not the same as a cleansing reaction, and it can be a scary experience for uninformed individuals. When we finally do things right, like cleanse, fast, and eat naturally, we will extract the toxins, poisons, and emotions that we had stored within our bodies and which were producing dis-ease. The healing crisis is like the completion of a cycle. The beginning of a dis-ease marks the beginning of a cycle in which a dis-ease inhabits and impairs the body to varying degrees, even after the acute phase of the illness has passed; the healing crisis is the ending of that cycle, freeing the body entirely from all influence of that dis-ease. When the healing crisis begins, we sometimes think that we are becoming worse instead of better. Without proper knowledge, some people become overly concerned or even fearful and then lose their common sense and stop doing the very things that are making them well. Then they often fall back into the habits that caused all their problems. This often occurs when friends or relatives are not informed about the benefits and actions of cleansing; well-intentioned relatives have persuaded many people to stop cleansing or fasting, even though it was the very best thing for their health. Therefore, it is important to understand the healing crisis. I've even seen parents sway a child away from following a program that would have saved the little one's life, and then watched their child die a miserable death.

The healing crisis is a great blessing. It is something we enthusiastically work toward. Dr. Bruce Fife, author of *The Healing Crisis,*[111] clearly explains that **removal of agents that cause dis-ease is the catalyst for both cleansing reactions and healing crises**. He points out that **most any harmless method** that strengthens the body's natural healing processes **can induce a healing crisis and/or cleansing reactions**. When it happens we should rejoice, knowing that we have eliminated more causes of dis-ease. It means that we have cleansed and purified our bodies from unwanted toxic waste which was poisoning the body, mind, and feelings, causing weakness and potential dis-ease. **After the healing crisis, we are *always* stronger than before, for the darkness is replaced with the light.**

This process is the exact opposite of what allopathic medicine does with its drugs. Drugs suppress and block, driving dis-ease into deeper levels or into other areas of the body. This temporarily changes the focus of

---

[111] Bruce Fife, N.D., *The Healing Crisis*, (Colorado Springs, CO: HealthWise Publications, 1997), pg 23.

symptoms and gives the false appearance of wellness. The truth is, the cause is still there and will erupt at a later time, possibly at a more critical time when we are less capable of coping with it. Cleansing, fasting, herbs, and changing attitudes **can bring the agents that cause dis-ease to the surface, and eliminate the cause of dis-ease and symptoms permanently.**

The experience of going through a healing crisis will seem very much like that of a dis-ease crisis. It is important to know the difference. If we are going through a healing crisis, we need to know that **it will soon pass** and that we are simply getting rid of the cause of dis-ease.

Joe Schecter of Tucson had accomplished about nine (9) Cleanses and started working on his gallbladder. One day he called. "Rich, how could it be that with all the cleansing I have done, that I could get asthma?"

"What do you mean?" I asked.

"I have all the symptoms – wheezing, coughing, and my breathing is shallow."

"Well," I said, "when did you have asthma before?"

"When I was in grade school."

"Expect it to last for about 3 days. If it lasts longer than that, call me."

I didn't hear from him for a two or three weeks, and when he came in to my office, I said, "How long did your asthma last?"

"My what? Oh, I forgot about that. Yeah, it went away in 3 days, just like you said."

My former wife had gone on the Cleanse three times in a seven-month period. After she completed her third Cleanse without having any cleansing reactions at all, she began to eat only raw fruits and vegetables. Then the cleansing reactions set in. She had every symptom of the walking pneumonia and bronchitis she had suffered in her childhood and early 20's. However, this time she rejoiced, for she knew that she was ridding herself of those ugly symptoms forever. For, the drugs her doctor had given her for those conditions suppressed the acute symptoms, but left her with wheezing, short breath, and heavy, stirred up congestion in her chest every single time she exercised.

With no thanks to the doctors, these 24 years of annoyance were about to be eliminated forever. After 10 days of telling herself and certain well-meaning individuals (who kept insisting that she had abused her body with "that fast") that she was just experiencing a valuable "healing crisis," her reward came. After that ten-day period, those symptoms disappeared and they never recurred, even when she was backpacking or playing tennis.

What is a Dis-ease Crisis?

A dis-ease crisis is the opposite of a healing crisis. Instead of getting better, one gets worse. A dis-ease crisis is a condition in which the dis-ease has developed to the point where it has become noticeable and uncomfortable. It has the potential of causing damage to metabolic function.

Note: The common cold is not a dis-ease crisis. It is a cleansing crisis. The good old American cold occurs after we have abused the body and the body dumps the overload of toxins. The cold is a *good* thing. **No one should ever attempt to stop it with drugs, but instead, should assist the body in eliminating its congestion through colonics or enemas, baths, herbal teas, and eating pure foods, such as vegetable juices and broths.** Allowing a cold to finish its cycle *ALWAYS* results in people feeling better and stronger. Stopping a cold with drugs *ALWAYS* results in future health problems.

How to Know if It is a Healing Crisis or a Dis-ease Crisis

As I stated above, the healing crisis and dis-ease crisis are opposites. The healing crisis is gaining health – eliminating dis-ease. It generally occurs after we have changed our diet and have begun taking good care of ourselves.

Dis-ease Crisis – The Curse of Bad Habits	Healing Crisis – The Blessing of Good Habits
*Comes with the warning of feeling not quite right.	*Usually comes with the warning of **feeling terrific the day before the crisis!**
*Caused by not taking care of the body, bad diet, stress, poor living habits.	*Caused by taking good care of the body, good diet, rest, good living habits.
***Body has become weaker and weaker – body vitality lowered.**	***Body vitality has become gradually stronger.**
*Processes of elimination are usually sluggish and incomplete.	*Elimination process is usually improved.
*The iris of the eye will usually show white areas **rising above** the iris level.	*The iris may show **white criss-crossed** "healing lines" **below** the normal iris level.

161

*These acute lines are usually **straight or parallel** to the trabeculae.	*These criss-crossing healing lines are **not parallel** to the trabeculae.
*Usually lasts three or seven days, but can last much longer.	*Usually lasts three days, but can last longer or shorter.
*Cannot remember the same problem occurring in the past	*Most people can recall a similar experience in the past.

Summary of Healing Crisis

No one has ever died from a healing crisis. The body never makes a mistake, and will not develop a healing crisis until the body is strong enough to handle it. **The day prior to a healing crisis we usually feel terrific.** Apparently, the body uses that energy to release something, for the crisis usually occurs after we hit the peak of energy; the next day is usually the day it begins. A healing crisis **usually** lasts only three days. However, it can last much longer, depending upon what is being released and how long it has been there, and also upon the vitality, the strength of the elimination organs, etc. **A person may need to go through many small healing crises before going through the final one.** As the cleansing or healing crises occur, they usually, but not always, follow a certain order. This order is called Hering's Law of Cure.

Note: For more details about the Healing Crisis, read our book *Dramatic Signs of Healing*, by Rich Anderson and G. Renee Getreu.

Hering's Law of Cure

1. Cures occur from within out,
2. From head down,
3. And in reverse order as dis-ease has developed.

Dr. Jensen wrote about two classic examples of healing crisis. Here is a good example of a healing crisis from his book, *Doctor-Patient Handbook*.[112]

*"Years ago I put a man, **almost blind and with heart trouble**, on a regular health routine of diet, exercise, and rest. About three months after starting treatment, I was called*

---

[112] Jensen, D.C., N.D., Ph.D., *Doctor-Patient Handbook*, (Escondido, CA: Bernard Jensen Publishing, 1976), pg. 54. For greater inspiration and more information, I suggest that everyone read Dr. Bernard Jensen's books.

*to his home. This man was having a heart crisis. His heart was beating so forcibly that his bed was moving on its casters. I knew this was a crisis and that he would come through all right. His crisis lasted twelve hours. **Almost immediately afterward he was able to read the newspaper for the first time in years. Later he was able to read fine print, and in about two months he attended a motion picture show.***"

Usually people forget what pain, injuries, or dis-ease they had in the past, until they're having a healing crisis. Then as they are experiencing the trouble, they remember, "This has happened before."

Another good example of a healing crisis comes from the *Doctor-Patient Handbook:*

*"... had an extreme curvature of the spine. As her healing progressed, she developed a severe 'cold', which lasted 15 or 20 days. It was necessary to assist her eliminative process with frequent eliminative treatments. During one of these treatments, she underwent the retracing of an experience she had gone through in an accident 15 years previously. For a few moments, she seemed to go all to pieces. **Her tongue swelled and she could hardly talk. For 15 minutes or so her body shook all over. She seemed to be in a critical condition,** but after this experience was over, the spinal tension disappeared, the curvature was decreased, and there was constant improvement in the spine throughout the following year. She felt better than she had in many years."*[113]

Following are two examples of men who went through many cleansing reactions, but had not yet experienced healing crisis. I assisted a man who had prostate cancer, and had decided to follow our Cleanse and diet regimen. This man, a pharmacist, was scheduled for an immediate operation, but his daughter persuaded him to use our cleansing program. He accomplished the Cleanse five (5) times during a three-month period! During this time, he experienced bloating, and fatigue on his first two cleanses. Then his energy improved tremendously. During his next cleanse, he developed skin rashes and depression. He endured one cleansing reaction after another. Coincidentally, a niece of his also had cancer, but she opted for chemotherapy. She called him once a week to tell him that he must have lost his mind – that following this cleansing and diet program

---

[113] Jensen, *ibid.*, pg. 54.

163

instead of choosing 'chemo' and surgery was insane! Then, during his third month she came to see him. She had to have help getting out of the car because she was so weak from the chemo. She was overweight and her breath was bad; her eyesight was dim, and she felt moody and depressed. Her skin was pale-gray, and all her hair had fallen out. When she rang the doorbell and he opened the door, she hardly recognized him. He had lost 30 pounds of fat, his skin was pink and radiant, his eyes were clear and sparkling, and his vitality revealed itself in each springy step he took. And to her utter astonishment, his joy overflowed as he shared his progress. He explained that the gastrointestinal disorder that he had suffered for years was gone; his irritable bowel syndrome and related toxemia were gone; his esophageal reflux condition that had become increasingly severe was gone; and his prostate cancer was reduced by 25%. And, by the way, this man, a pharmacist, does recommend cleansing!

Another man, who suffered from liver cancer and cirrhosis of the liver, came to see me. In this condition, red blood cells have the shape of stars, and severe weakness is accompanied by edema, depression, obesity, and pain. This man's pain was so severe that drugs had no effect upon him, and the doctors gave up on him. He began cleansing immediately and took a coffee colonic or enemas daily. Within 24 hours his pain greatly subsided and after the fourth day, 100% of his pain was gone. Within two weeks, he had no more edema and his energy increased. A registered nurse was assisting him, and she had witnessed all these changes. After she viewed the improvements in his blood, she broke down and wept. She was deeply moved by the incredible improvements she saw in him, but she was struck with a terrible grief for the millions of people under the guidance of well-intentioned medical doctors, people whom she knows will never experience the incredible benefits of detoxification. Did this man go through cleansing reactions? Most certainly! Almost every day. But within 30 days, he no longer needed his cane, his weight was normal, his depression was nearly gone. His mind was also clear again, and he was planning to go back to work!

Allowing the body to eliminate toxins naturally requires a sound understanding of both cleansing reactions and the healing crisis. The next step is to learn what actions will best facilitate complete cleansing at the times cleansing reactions or healing crises arise, **for you never, ever, want to stop a healing crisis.**

The Role of the Liver and Other Organs in Cleansing Reactions

Generally speaking, people who never experience a cleansing reaction and feel good throughout all phases of cleansing have a strong healthy liver. Those who experience cleansing reactions, especially during the Mildest or Gentle Phases, have a very weak liver. Other organs can be associated with cleansing reactions, especially the kidneys, but the liver is the primary organ to filter out toxins from the blood. **If the liver is unable to handle the toxins, then a cleansing reaction will occur.** Therefore, I recommend that all those who have experienced cleansing reactions during cleansing, become serious about working on cleansing and strengthening the liver after they have completed at least one cleanse, **for the first step in cleansing and strengthening the liver is to cleanse the liver's primary source of toxicity – the bowel.**[114]

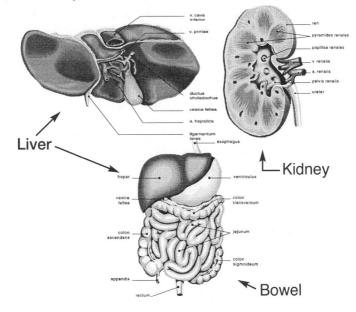

A cleansing reaction may occur any time the body is releasing toxins faster than it is able to eliminate them and faster than the liver can efficiently handle. For instance, toxins may be released into the intestine when a piece of mucoid plaque, which may have been stockpiling toxins, breaks loose. Some of these toxins may be absorbed back into the portal

---

[114] For more information about liver cleansing and strenghtening the liver, read my booklet *The Liver: The Vital Organ*, available through Christobe Publishing. (503) 926-8855.

veins, which go directly to the liver. **Do you know what the liver does to get rid of toxins?** Although, there are some toxins that the liver can convert to non-toxins, most toxins are released from the liver via the gall juices. The gall juices carry the toxins into the duodenum and then down through the alimentary canal and out through a bowel movement. Guess what happens when a person is constipated? Yes, the bowel can reabsorb the toxins, which forces them to reenter the liver again. **Therefore, the very first step that all doctors and healers should take is to eliminate constipation.** And another very important thing we can do is to use psyllium-bentonite shakes in proper timing on a cleanse, for these shakes absorb toxins, binding them until the bowel removes the mass out of the body.

It should by now be obvious that all cleansing reactions – including headaches, aching muscles or joints, fever, sweating, body odor, rashes, bad breath, loss of appetite, sleepiness, and weakness or exhaustion – are indications that one's diet and/or lifestyle has been dis-ease producing, resulting in ineffective digestion, poor bowel function, and liver weakness. Further cleansing reactions, such as **nausea, vomiting and diarrhea,** occur when extreme toxins, pathogenic bacteria, yeast, parasites, or acids are still in the stomach and intestines. These reactions prove beyond doubt that one has been accumulating substance that causes dis-ease to harmful levels. It also indicates that intestinal cleansing is way past due. Cleansing should, ideally, have been accomplished years in advance of these conditions, thus preventing their development. Cleansing reactions also indicate that cleansing needs to be continued, for if these symptom-causing toxins are not removed, then serious, even life-threatening, diseases are likely to develop.

Basic Steps to Relieve Cleansing Reactions

While cleansing, we can assist the body in its effort to eliminate this excess toxicity in several ways. Taking these basic steps relieves most cleansing reactions fairly quickly, that is, within a few minutes to a few hours.

1. **Drink extra water.** Sometimes elimination slows down because a person is not drinking enough water. Without water the body has no medium to use for removing toxins. Make sure you are taking in plenty of water.
2. If colonics or enemas do not produce the desired effect, then **a coffee colonic or enema** may prove helpful, as it will cause the liver to dump toxicity out through the bile. Instructions for a coffee colonic or enema may be found in Chapter 13. It is

estimated that even when cleansing reactions are severe, such as intense headaches and extreme weakness, that between 80% and 90% of people cleansing can eliminate 90% to 100% of their symptoms by using the coffee enema. These outstanding results from the coffee enema confirm that **the principal cause of these undesirable symptoms was a weak liver.**

3. **Take extra amounts of organic alkalizing minerals.** The body requires alkalizing electrolyte minerals to buffer the toxic acids that must be removed. Without enough electrolyte minerals, the body is unable to remove acid toxins, and these acids in circulation weaken the body. In addition, extra alkalizing minerals should always be taken any time someone takes a coffee colonic or enema, because the body uses electrolytes to produce new bile.

4. **Take pure-water colonics or enemas – preferably colonics.** If colonics are unavailable, I recommend using at least three enema bags (2 quarts each) of water or more, or at least until the water comes out fairly clear. (Each bag of water should be eliminated before taking in the next bag.) Instructions for how to take an enema are found in Chapter 13.

Specific and Additional Steps to Relieve Specific Cleansing Reactions

> **Note:** Always *begin* with the basic steps discussed above. The following offers tips for specific types of reactions. **LISTEN TO YOUR BODY. BE GENTLE WITH YOURSELF!** And always ask your inner self, "Should I do this now?" or, "Is this right for me?"

Constipation
(During a cleanse)

❑ Check to be sure you are taking the proper amount of psyllium in the shake. The maximum amount should be two (2) slightly rounded **tea**spoons – **NOT TABLE**spoons.

❑ Gradually increase amount of cleansing herb formulas.

❑ Take a colonic or enema to get things moving.

❑ Take more electrolyte minerals – from broth, juices, and supplements – to correct pH.

❑ Take your shake **without** bentonite for one (1) day.

❏ Take more of the less acid probiotic, three (3) times a day for five (5) days.
❏ Make sure you are getting at least four (4) quarts of liquid daily.

(After a cleanse)
❏ Drink two 16-ounce glasses of water each morning, with fresh lemon juice.
❏ Take more of the less acid-forming, general-use probiotic, three (3) to four (4) times a day for five to seven (5-7) days.
❏ Drink a shake **without** bentonite first thing in the morning.
❏ Take an herbal laxative desgined to strengthen perastalsis, one and one-half hours after the shake.

```
Note: Constipation may be associated with[115]:
     ♦   Lack of friendly bacteria
     ♦   Mucoid plaque
     ♦   Weak liver
     ♦   Pathogenic bacteria, parasites, yeast
     ♦   Hormonal imbalance
     ♦   Weak peristaltic muscles
     ♦   Lack of fiber
     ♦   Prolonged mineral depletion
     ♦   Suppressed emotions
```

Diarrhea
❏ Decrease the amount of cleansing herb formulas for a day or two.
❏ Add my special herbal aid formula, along with a reduced dose of my regular cleansing herb Formula #1, for a more gentle laxative effect.
❏ Increase the amount of bentonite and/or psyllium in the shake.
❏ Take the organic electrolyte mineral supplement.
❏ Discontinue cayenne, if using it. May introduce it again slowly after the diarrhea is gone.
❏ If diarrhea is severe, take one (1) teaspoon of L-Glutamine, three (3) times daily
❏ Take extra green drinks and carrot juice to provide extra electrolyte minerals.

---

[115] As noted on page 20, the "diamond bullets" indicate warning points.

Headaches

Take a colema, colonic, or enemas until the water circulating back out is fairly clear. If these procedures do not relieve the pain, a coffee enema usually will.

Nausea

- [ ] Take a psyllium-bentonite shake with extra bentonite to help absorb more toxins.
- [ ] Take a thorough colonic or enema, usually with two to three (2-3) consecutive bags of water, or until the water comes out fairly clear.
- [ ] Drink peppermint or ginger tea.
- [ ] When nausea is caused by a microorganism, one-quarter (1/4) teaspoon of my more acid-forming probiotic formula usually eliminates the problem within a few minutes or hours.
- [ ] If you feel sick shortly after taking the herbs, try taking them one at a time in five-minute intervals.
- [ ] Go back to an earlier phase, to give your body more time to detox at a slower rate.
- [ ] If you suspect parasites, and nothing else relieves the nausea to a level that you can endure, stop the Cleanse and follow the parasite program first. Then return to the Cleanse. Most people who have followed this course did not experience further nausea when they began the Cleanse again.
- [ ] Take a coffee enema to relieve the liver.

Vomiting

- [ ] Let the body vomit. Drink peppermint tea afterwards.
- [ ] If vomiting persists, take a psyllium-bentonite shake with two to three (2-3) times the normal amount of bentonite.
- [ ] If the above fails, and vomiting is very severe and causing dry heaves every few minutes, it is likely caused by parasites, bacteria, or acids. Sipping on bentonite water every few minutes has been effective within 5 to 10 minutes: Add approximately one to four (1-4) tablespoons of bentonite to four to ten (4-10) ounces of water, stir, and sip slowly.
- [ ] If it still persists, take L. glutamine.
- [ ] After vomiting stops, take organic electrolyte mineral supplements to help replace the electrolytes that are lost during vomiting.
- [ ] If vomiting persists after the above, call my office.

> **Note**: In 13 years, we have heard of two or three people who appeared to have an allergy to psyllium. Indicators would be: 1) uncontrolled vomiting *immediately* after intake, and 2) nausea for several hours after. I have developed an alternative bulking agent formula for such cases.

Sleepiness, Weakness, or Exhaustion

This may occur for two reasons during the Cleanse:
1. The body is using all of its energy to cleanse and rejuvenate, OR
2. Organs such as the liver and kidneys may be weak and sluggish because of excessive toxins.

The solution I recommend is to either:
1. Have a colonic or enema to release more toxic debris, or
2. Take a coffee enema to release toxins from the liver.

Bloating and Gas

Bloating may be caused by gas. Gas will sometimes follow a release of plaque as unfriendly bacteria and/or parasites, which had been hidden beneath the plaque, are briefly unconfined before elimination. Continued cleansing eventually eliminates the cause.

CHAPTER 13

HOW TO TAKE AN ENEMA

The First Recorded Directions on How to Take an Enema

"Think not that it is sufficient that the angel of water embrace you outwards only. I tell you truly, the uncleanness within is greater by much than the uncleanness without. **And he, who cleanses himself without, but within remains unclean, is like to tombs that outwards are painted fair, but are within full of all manner of horrible uncleanness and abominations.**

Seek, therefore, a large trailing gourd, having a stalk the length of a man; take out its innards and fill it with water from the river, which the sun has warmed. Hang it upon a branch of a tree, and kneel upon the ground before the angel of water, and suffer the end of the stalk of the trailing gourd to enter your hinder parts [so] that the water may flow through all your bowels. Afterwards rest kneeling on the ground before the angel of water **that he will free your body from every uncleanness and dis-ease.** *Then let the water run out from your body, that it may carry away from within all the unclean and evil-smelling things of Satan.* **And you shall see with your eyes and smell with your nose all the abominations and uncleanness which defiled the temple of your body; even all the sins which abode in your body, tormenting you with all manner of pains."**[116]

---

[116] John (Disciple of Jesus Christ) recorded these words of Jesus. See Edmund Bordeaux Szekely, ed., *Gospel of Peace of Jesus Christ*, as recorded by John, the Disciple of Christ (Nelson, B.C., Canada: International Biogenic Society, 1981.)

Nothing Gives Relief as Does an Enema

Learn to appreciate and enjoy enemas. Nothing short of Divine Intervention (also known as miracles) can come to your rescue faster to relieve you of headaches, constipation, pressure, various pains, gas and massive accumulations of toxic mucus, pus, and poisonous waste – which all contribute towards dis-ease.

Some people are downright afraid to take enemas. This is generally due to either embarrassment or lack of knowledge. **Anything this good for you should not be embarrassing.** Taking enemas is wise and intelligent. They are fully constructive, lifting you to a higher level of existence through purification. If you are going to be embarrassed, consider being embarrassed by the things you do which are destructive to your Temple – like drinking alcoholic beverages, coffee, and pop; eating meat, sugar, and dairy products; eating more than you need; swearing; or being overweight.

On the other hand, you simply may not know *how* to take an enema. Don't let that stop you; it's easy to learn. Be brave! Consider it a new dimension of living yet to be explored. A vast, new frontier of experience awaits you! I guarantee you it will become the most enjoyable part of the Cleanse – seeing the results of your efforts coming out of you in vivid living color!

When on the Cleanse, taking enemas twice daily will usually help a person rid himself of an extra ten feet of mucoid layers in a seven-day period. I know a friend who refused to take enemas during the Cleanse. Being an herbalist, he figured that if he took extra *cascara sagrada* he could keep things moving and avoid enemas completely. But there were times when he did not feel good – a clear indication that toxic substance was being stirred up and needed to be released. He would have had relief had he taken an enema. The next time he went on the Cleanse, he decided to use the enemas. He overcame his aversion to them very quickly when he saw the benefits. His cleansing went much easier and he now recommends enemas to everyone doing the Cleanse.

Most toxic people I have seen go on this Cleanse without taking enemas have had a worse-than-average experience. When you become really miserable and your friend, Mr. Pain, brings you to your senses, your silly embarrassment or lack of knowledge will be something you will want to conquer, instead of letting it conquer you.

Note: Enemas are terrific, but if you need something even more effective, a colonic usually brings immense relief.

Instructions and Equipment Needed

I recommend a **douche bag** instead of the enema/hot water bags you find in the drug stores. The point is that you want a bag that is open at the top so you can easily refill it and keep it clean. Douche bags are also easier and faster to use and less expensive. Olive oil or an ointment that contains natural herbs and beeswax is the best lubricant to place on the injection tip for easy insertion. A dab of the same lubricant is also placed on the anus. This combination makes for easy injection. Any kind of salad oil is okay, but olive oil is very healing and purifying – in addition to being good for most rashes.

It is helpful to use a gallon jug to fill the douche bag with water or herbal tea. You can use any size of container, but the gallon jug makes it easier and faster to use.

What to Use for Enema Liquid

Most of the time, I use an herbal tea, but you can use plain old tap water. But, it must be free of contaminants, including chlorine and fluoride. Obviously, we would not use tap water in most areas of our country. Where I live, the water is just about as pure as it gets. In Chicago, I wouldn't even consider it. You must also be careful with well water; in many areas of the country, the well water is highly contaminated. Distilled water is best; purified water of high quality is fine. The following herbs make excellent enemas:

- ❑ *CATNIP* has a soothing effect on the body. It is good for energy, improves circulation, and is excellent for colds, fever, and gas. Children or those who have trouble taking enemas may especially benefit from catnip.
- ❑ *BURDOCK ROOT* is one of the best blood purifiers you'll find; it is the best herb for skin; it improves kidney action, helping to eliminate calcium deposits; and it assists the liver in removing toxins.
- ❑ *YARROW* is one of the bitter herbs; it is good for the liver, stomach, and glands. A blood purifier, it opens the pores of the skin (the body's largest elimination organ) for rapid elimination. It is good for colds, cramps, fever, and flu; and also good for infusion in a healing bath.
- ❑ *RED RASPBERRY* is excellent for all kinds of gynecologic problems. High in iron, it is good for the eyes and for elimination; it is very nutritious.

173

- **KIDNEY TEA** is a combination of herbs for the kidneys and urinary system. I made these into a wonderful formula that I use in almost every enema I take.
- **WILD CHERRY BARK** is very useful for those do not eliminate their enema water easily. Make a tea using one (1) teaspoon in a quart of water, and add it to approximately one and one-half (1-1/2) gallons of enema water.
- **OTHER EXCELLENT ENEMA HERBS** include blessed thistle, hyssop, elderflower, mullein, and dandelion.

Temperature of Enema Liquid

I prefer the liquid to be right at body temperature. If it is too warm the muscles will temporarily weaken, and this prevents the water from rushing back out, which you want it to do. The muscles will stay strong with liquid that is at or slightly below body temperature.

To awaken and bring strength to the peristaltic muscles in the colon, use cooler or cold water for your last half-gallon of enema liquid (it is best to do this after you feel you've removed all of the loose matter out of the colon with a gallon of water at body temperature first). You will feel a wonderful sensation down in the colon that will strengthen the whole lower abdomen.

Injection Procedure

Place the empty enema bag on the shower or bathroom door handle, or on the towel rack. This is a comfortable height. After you get used to enemas, feel free to hang the bag higher. However, the higher you hang the bag, the more pressure there is, making the liquid flow out faster. (However, you can control the flow with the enema bag shut-off valve, which is about two inches from the tip.) Then fill it from your gallon bottle.

Note: When putting liquid in the enema bag, be sure the valve is shut. After you've sprayed your feet and clean bathroom with an herbal-tea enema the first time, you won't have to remind yourself of this anymore!

Put the lubricant on the enema tip and on the anus. Place the tip over the toilet, sink, or bathtub, or into the gallon jug you poured from, and open the valve, allowing the liquid to flow until the air bubbles are removed from the tube. Then shut the valve, get into position and insert. After insertion, open the valve gradually, allowing the liquid to flow up the colon slowly until you get used to it. Always keep your hand on the valve for quick shut-off when needed and to keep the tip from slipping out.

Position for the Enema

Some people prefer lying on the back; this way they are in a good position to be comfortable and massage the colon. I like to be on my knees with my head on a towel; it feels like the liquid flows in easier and more easily reaches all areas of the colon than when I'm on my back. Always massage the abdomen while in that position and before getting up to eliminate, so that much more debris will be removed.

Starting with the descending colon (left side of the lower abdomen), gently massage upwards to the transverse colon (found just behind the lower rib cage, unless you have a prolapsus), and then down the ascending colon (right side). Work it well – get the liquid all the way down to the ileocecal. If you aren't sure where all these parts of the colon are, just massage the heck out of your lower abdomen, moving from the lower left, up the left side, across just below the ribs, and down the right side. Then go to the toilet and release! Be prepared to be amazed and astounded at what you will eliminate. Now you will begin to enjoy enemas. Keep in mind that, depending on your pre-cleanse preparation, you may not get any of the "real stuff" out until your fourth or fifth day.

At times, when the liquid has difficulty flowing up into the colon, it helps considerably to take deep breaths – all the way in and all the way out. This changes the pressure in the abdomen area and makes it easier for the liquid to pass through.

Amount of Liquid

When you first begin the enema, you may only get a cup or so of liquid in, depending upon how compacted you are. That's okay, don't force it. As soon as the pressure gets uncomfortable, shut off the valve. Try to work the liquid past the congestion by massaging as indicated above; then add more liquid; you will know when it's too much. Then evacuate. You should pass some blockages. Let it all out, and then repeat the procedure. This time you will get more liquid in. Although you may never reach it, make a goal of continuing the procedure until all chunks stop coming out. Who would want putrefying toxic garbage in their bodies even a second

175

longer than absolutely necessary? I recommend going through two or more gallons. If you are pressed for time, remember that a shorter enema is infinitely better than no enema. And you'll be a *lot* more comfortable wherever you're going if you take that extra time for your enema before you go.

I would recommend you take the enemas first thing in the morning and at five or six in the evening. If you take one just before bed, you may have to get up during the night, since liquid is often left in the colon, and gradually seeps into the bladder, until pretty soon you will need to awake to eliminate.

If you already have to get up several times during the night, try chewing juniper berries. This will help break up uric acid deposits and clean the urinary system. It will also help relax the bladder. After taking juniper for a day or two, you will experience how much it can assist you in sleeping through the night. Using juniper tea can make that happen even sooner. You can also use an herbal formula that contains gravel root, juniper berries, uva ursi leaf, burdock root, hydrangea root, parsley leaf, marshmallow root, ginger root, and lobelia leaf. I created a formula with these herbs, which I personally use. I can tell you, it produces wonderful results. If a man has a slow urine flow and uses this formula without results, then he may have a prostate enlargement. Using a quality tincture of saw palmetto should relieve the problem within a few days. If it fails to do this, either it was a poor-quality tincture or he may have a serious prostate problem and should plan on doing some serious cleansing and rebuilding.

The Coffee Enema

The following is based upon Dr. Gerson's work. More information is available in his book, *A Cancer Therapy: Results of Fifty Cases.*

For reducing pain of the worst kind or for eliminating extreme toxic side effects produced by drugs or other toxins affecting the liver, there is nothing more effective than a coffee enema. The liver must handle most of the poisons and other toxins that have found their way into the liver, and a coffee enema is the fastest known method of reducing liver toxicity.

Coffee enemas help remove toxins from the liver quickly and safely. They often provide quick relief when fatigued, sleepy, or headachy, or for just plain malaise. They help reduce or eliminate spasms, precordial (heart, throat, chest) pain, and difficulties resulting from the sudden withdrawal of all intoxicating substances. They also help eliminate headaches caused by coffee withdrawal. Chronic and degenerative dis-eases

176

are usually associated with a faltering liver, a condition that is often associated with liver toxicity; and coffee enemas have been effective in purging the liver of toxins that diminish liver function.

A coffee enema, when used properly, causes the liver to produce more bile and open the bile ducts. This causes the bile to quickly flow out of the liver. During this process, a toxic liver can dump many of its toxicants into the bile, thus getting rid of them in just a few minutes. This can give great relief to all parts of the body, especially the liver. It can easily make the difference between someone feeling so poorly that he or she has to lie down, or feeling well enough to keep active; and in some cases, it can make the difference between life and death.

In extremely toxic individuals, the bile may contain poisons that can cause spasms in the duodenum and small intestines. In rare cases, it is possible, during these times, that some bile may flow into the stomach, which can cause nausea, or vomiting of bile. This usually occurs when the colon has not been emptied prior to using the coffee enema. Therefore, it is important to empty the colon with enemas or colonics before doing a coffee enema. If nausea does occur, drink large amounts of peppermint tea to help wash the bile from the stomach.

There are two other reasons why we should empty the colon prior to using the coffee enema: 1) An empty colon allows the coffee to remain in the colon for the allotted time; and 2) colonics or enemas eliminate colonic toxicity that could "hitchhike" with the coffee and enter the liver. Obviously, we never want this to occur. Therefore, it is important to always flush out the colon before using the coffee enema.

Drinking a cup of coffee has an entirely different effect, one that is detrimental to the body. Drinking coffee causes the following problems: increased reflex response, low blood pressure, increased heart rate, insomnia, constipation, heart palpitation, over-stimulation of the adrenals, stomach irritation, and toxic residues in the body. A coffee enema when done properly will not produce these effects. In fact, a coffee enema will completely eliminate withdrawals associated with the ceasing of habitual coffee drinking.

WARNING: Great care should be used if taking coffee enemas when water fasting. Coffee enemas cause bile to be excreted from the liver. The bile contains many valuable mineral salts, the loss of which can be very harmful, if they are not replenished. People using one or more coffee enemas per day must be on a good diet of broths and fresh juices or a natural electrolyte minerals supplement such as my main alkalizing supplement, to assure the replenishing of these mineral salts.

177

During intestinal cleansing, one coffee enema daily may be helpful as long as pH tests were passed before starting to cleanse. Otherwise, the drinking of fresh juices, especially carrot, beet, and celery juice, are highly recommended. Taking alkalizing minerals (electrolyte minerals from food sources only) will also help to replenish the bile salts lost through coffee enemas.

In serious cases of cancer, especially when pain is being experienced, it may be necessary to perform a coffee enema every six hours, night and day – in the most serious cases, every hour. A coffee enema may be helpful once a day for about 7 days during cleansing. Otherwise it should be used only when one is feeling bad – having headaches, etc. Remember, each person needs to choose what is best for his or her body.

Preparing the Coffee Enema

Use three (3) tablespoons of ground coffee (organically grown coffee is essential) to one (1) quart of water (preferably distilled). Boil for three (3) minutes, and then simmer for 20 minutes. Strain and cool to body temperature. Prepare only the amount to be used that day; do not store overnight.

Important! Lie down on your right side, with both legs drawn close to the abdomen. Deep breathing is recommended to draw the greatest amount of fluid into the necessary parts of the colon. It also helps to let all the air out of the lungs and suck the abdomen in and out while in this position.

The fluid should be retained for 15 minutes. It helps to have a clock in clear view. It may also help to have something to read while the water is flowing in and being retained. Dr. Gerson found that all the caffeine is absorbed from the fluid in 10 to 12 minutes. The caffeine goes through the hemorrhoidal veins directly into the portal veins and then into the liver, causing the effects already described.

Note: It is a very good idea to be taking at least two psyllium-bentonite shakes daily to help absorb the toxins that are released from the bile into the small intestine by the coffee enema.

Additional Note: For thorough liver purification, it is also suggested to follow the liver program in my booklet, *The Liver: The Vital Organ.* Also, you should be on the Mildest Phase, as indicated in the booklet. Besides the herbs indicated in the booklet, take the Blood Purifying formula.

Peppermint Tea Preparation

For nausea, which a few may experience when doing a coffee enema, drinking peppermint tea can help.

Add one (1) tablespoon of dried peppermint leaves to two (2) cups (one pint) of boiling water (preferably distilled water). Let it lightly simmer for five (5) minutes, and strain before drinking.

CHAPTER 14

SECRETS OF GOOD HEALTH

*"There is no such thing as an incurable dis-ease –
only people who make wrong choices.*

*Did you know that there has never been a dis-ease
that someone hasn't conquered?"*

– Rich Anderson, N.D., N.M.D.

Eating Devitalized Foods

Our bodies are designed to partake of raw foods only. Notice that our Creator did not issue stoves or ovens to any animal, bird, fish, or human. Notice also that no creature of God uses refrigerators or freezers, except for those cocky humans. And, while we're on the subject, notice that no animal in its right mind smokes cigarettes, drinks alcohol, or adds unnatural chemicals to its food, air, or water. Only those who are out of balance with Nature do these cock-eyed, self-destructive things. To continue, foods that have been cooked, frozen, canned, or processed are dead foods, and are not fit for human, or animal, consumption. I propose that the true definition of a food is as follows: a substance that nourishes or fuels the body with life-giving forces (i.e. life force, vitamins, minerals, enzymes, amino acids, etc.), without injury to its normal functions, thereby strengthening, energizing, and maintaining it. Food is not simply something one puts in the mouth, chews, and swallows. Food should not deplete or rob the body of its needed essence or harm it in any way. Dead or dying foods take an enormous toll on the body.

Facts About What Cooked, Frozen, Canned, and Processed Foods Really Do

- ❑ provide deficient levels of vitamins
- ❑ create toxins and acids
- ❑ drain the life force from the body
- ❑ poison the liver and bloodstream

- ❏ clog the body's lymph system
- ❏ drain the body's enzyme reserve
- ❏ overwork and clog the elimination systems
- ❏ strain the glandular system
- ❏ overwork the digestive system and liver
- ❏ cause stress, congestion, and mucus
- ❏ produce the ideal environment for parasites and other unnatural pathogens

In a few years, the scientific world will be forced to announce that the natural food for man is raw fruits, raw vegetables, sprouted seeds, grains, legumes, nuts, and herbs. For those who use the Bible as an authority, reading Genesis and Ezekiel may prove enlightening.[117] Ah yes, I know some would say that there are other examples of biblical contradictions to these passages, and therefore they cannot be fully relied upon as infallible Divine direction. Biblical interpretations aside, it is not my intent to criticize those who rationalize their poor eating habits, but to encourage them to break out of those habits, which are making them sick and prematurely old. Investigation of the anatomy of the human body with particular attention to the digestive processes proves, beyond any doubt, what we should and should not eat. **When we eat unnatural foods, we are literally poisoning ourselves.** Sugar, pop, coffee, alcohol, fried foods, preservatives, and all other chemicals in food are poisons. Pasteurized dairy products, meat, cooked foods, and wheat are poisonous to most people and overwork the body into dis-ease.

Avoid Dairy Products

Pasteurized cow's milk in any form is the most mucus-forming of all so-called foods. Cow's milk is NOT the same as human milk. It is unnatural to man. Its imbalanced minerals create an unfavorable response in the body. Because it contains too much phosphorous, it is actually a calcium-deficient substance, which is why they add Vitamin D to milk – to help cloak the calcium loss.[118] When pasteurized, cow's milk becomes a poison. **Even a calf will die in three to six months when fed only**

---

[117] See Genesis 1:29: "And God said, Behold, I have given you every herb-bearing seed, which is upon the face of all the earth, and every tree, in which is the fruit of a tree yielding seed; to you it shall be for meat." Also see, Ezekiel 47:12: "...and the fruit thereof shall be for meat, and the leaf thereof for medicine."

[118] Vitamin D is known to enhance calcium absorption. If milk were a good source of calcium, why would dairy companies go to the extra expense of adding Vitamin D to their milk?

pasteurized milk. Do you think human children can live any better on pasteurized cow's milk than the calf for which the milk was originally designed?

Not only that, but more than 50% of Americans are allergic to dairy products, mainly because they lack the lactase enzyme. These facts and more are explained in more detail in my book *Cleanse & Purify Thyself,* Book 2. It tells of the clinical studies that prove that cow's milk is a negative source of calcium and actually harmful to the body. Those who must use dairy products should use those made with *raw* goat's milk, since it is nearer to human milk and much less mucus-forming.

Avoid Meat

The digestive system of the meat-eating animal is completely different from that of a human being. Its entire digestive tract is only twelve feet long compared to almost 30 feet in a human being. The meat eater's digestion requires ten times more hydrochloric acid than can be provided by the human body, and most people today are unable to produce even normal levels of hydrochloric acid. Many early peoples, including the Essene Hebrews, Buddhists, some groups of Hindus, and others were vegetarian. In addition to the Bible passages in Genesis and Ezekiel that I have already mentioned, Saint Paul, in Romans 14:21, said, "*It is good not to eat flesh.*" Romans: 14:21

In *The Gospel of the Perfect Life*, Jesus is recorded as saying:

"I am come to end the sacrifices and feasts of blood, and if ye cease not offering and eating of flesh and blood, the wrath of God shall not cease from you, even as it came to your fathers in the wilderness, who lusted for flesh, and they ate to their content, and were filled with rottenness, and the plaque consumed them."[19]

When we realize that the epidemics of heart dis-ease and cancer currently take the lives of more than 65% of the American population, we may consider that the above words were a prophecy that has come true.

Science has long supported the consumption of meat, but in the last few decades much has been learned and science can no longer offer that support, for to do so would now be a lie. The facts are so

---

[19] *Gospel of the Perfect Life*, (Mt. Shasta, CA: Christobe Publishing, projected publication 2001), Chapter 21:8.

overwhelming that the practice of eating of animal flesh is doomed as the age of enlightened people is ushered in. One day mankind will look back in horror at the carnivorous habits of its predecessors. The habit of eating meat will appear barbaric and disgusting to future man, as the eating of cat and dog meat now seems to the average American.

Note: Most American vegetarians were once meat eaters, and even after many years, they carry old, dead meat or its toxins in their intestinal tracts. It requires serious cleansing to get rid of it. Lifelong vegetarians have a tremendous advantage, even if they eat poorly, as many do.

Many people have asked me, "Where do you get your protein?" I answer, "From watermelon, and my wife gets hers from lettuce." Protein is in every single food you eat except oils. The protein myth was created to further a brainwashing program promoted by the meat and dairy industries. Their facts were based upon unreliable data. For an example, the medical suggestions for the amounts of protein needed for human consumption is based upon rats, not humans. A baby rat doubles its weight in just a few days drinking its mother's milk, which is about 15% protein. Human babies double their weight in about 180 days, drinking human mother's milk, which has about 2% or 3% protein. Yet the suggested daily protein is based upon rats. Does this make any "cents?" No! It makes *dollars*, billions of dollars, for it keeps the dis-ease and dairy industry highly profitable. Even suggestions regarding the essential and nonessential amino acids were also based upon a study of rats, not humans. Really, someone should tell some of these researchers that there is a vast difference between rats and humans, at least most humans.[120] But then again, maybe these *researchers* were rats.

Where does a cow get its protein? Are cows, from whence most meat eaters derive their proteins, protein deficient? They're strict vegetarians, at least a few of them still are.[121] I say, "Why settle for *used* protein? Why not get it directly from the same source as does a cow – the vegetable kingdom."

---

[120] Maurice E. Shils and Vernon R. Young, *Modern Nutrition in Health and Dis-ease*, 7th Edition, (Philadelphia, PA: Lea & Febiger, 1988), pg. 5, 29. Also, W. C. Rose, *Physiology Review*, 1938; Vol. 18, pg. 109-136.

[121] Many of the cattle in America are now cannibals, thanks to feed companies that mix dead animals, including beef, with cattle feed. It was found that when cattle injested meat they produced much more milk, and gained significantly more weight. It has a horrible repercussion however; it creates Mad Cow's Dis-ease. Yes, Mad Cow's Dis-ease has entered America. This has been covered up, but is a reality. Check the web for more information.

I was flying from L.A. to Seattle one day and was seated next to a young German woman. When the intercom asked Rich Anderson to identify himself, I pushed the button. The lady asked me what it was about and I explained that it was for my vegetarian meal. She said she ate meat and asked why I didn't. I said, "I love animals." (Lots easier than going into mucoid-fecal-matter conversation and, besides, it's true.) And as she took a bite of meat from her plate, she said, "So do I!" I looked at her in disbelief and said, "Are you sure?" She got the message and for several minutes just sat there looking stunned. I suppose other people love animals in different ways – some love them to eat; others just love them.

True Facts About Meat

- ❏ Study after study reveals that meat eaters develop much more dis-ease than vegetarians do. Meat eaters have far more osteoporosis, arthritis, bone dis-ease, diabetes, heart dis-ease, asthma, liver and kidney problems, as well as cancer, AIDS, and heart dis-ease, etc.[122]
- ❏ In 1961, the *Journal of the American Medical Association* reported that a vegetarian diet can prevent 90-97% of heart dis-eases. Hundreds of clinical studies substantiate these facts.
- ❏ Studies reveal 59% less cancer among people who eat small amounts of meat, compared to average meat eaters. These figures would be even more impressive if compared to vegetarians, and especially lifelong vegetarians.
- ❏ Scotland has the highest rate of bowel cancer in the world, and the Scottish people eat 20% more meat than the English.
- ❏ During World War I, Norway and Denmark could not obtain meat. Their death rates dropped 17% and then returned to normal after they returned to their meat diets.
- ❏ The kidneys of the meat eater must work three times harder than the kidneys of the vegetarian.
- ❏ The American National Institute of Health, in a study of 50,000 vegetarians, found that they live longer, have far less heart dis-ease, and have a much lower cancer rate compared to meat eaters.[123]

---

[122] M. L. Burr; and P. M. Sweetnam, "Vegetarianism, Dietary Fiber, and Mortality," *American Journal of Clinical Nutrition*, 1982; Nov.; Vol. 36, pg. 873-877.

[123] Note: Most American vegetarians were once meat eaters and, even after many years on a vegetarian diet, they still carry old, dead meat or its toxins in their bodies. It takes serious cleansing to remove it. Lifelong

- Studies show that vegetarians are stronger, more agile, have greater endurance, and recover from fatigue faster than meat eaters.
- A Yale University study revealed that vegetarians have nearly twice the stamina of meat eaters.[124]
- Cornell University announced through major newspapers in May of 1990, "Humans are natural vegetarians." The report said, "Animal foods, in general, are not really helpful and we need to get away from eating them."
- World starvation is strongly connected to meat-eating habits. If Americans stopped feeding grain to cattle, the excess grain could feed 500 million people, not to mention the land that could be used to grow food instead of being used for grazing cattle.
- In England, vegetarians pay less for life insurance.

How the Manipulators Have Dulled the Minds of Nations, and How to Avoid Manipulation

And what dulls the mind? The two most important factors are the consuming of white sugar and the eating of meat. A third factor may be fluoride in drinking water and toothpaste.

And how do we, personally, weaken our minds? By allowing ourselves to dwell in judgment and opinionism, for this opens us up to negative thinking. It repels love and replaces it with all sorts of dark thoughts and feelings. I know that these ideas may be a bit of a stretch for some readers to accept. Yet a thorough inquiry will reveal that it isn't just my opinion, it's a fact.

---

vegetarians have a tremendous advantage, even if they eat poorly, as many do. When this study was made, most of the vegetarians ate large amounts of meat substitutes, the highly processed soy products, which are detrimental to the human body.

[124] In this study, meat-eating college athletes were compared to vegetarian non-athletes – not a fair study, by any means, yet the vegetarians impressed everyone.

Is It Easy to Suddenly Become a "Raw-fooder"?

For some, perhaps; I admit it hasn't been easy for me. In fact, I still am not a complete raw-fooder; although I have periods when I do eat only raw food. I also have periods, especially when I am traveling, when I eat way too much cooked food. But, I at least know what to do about it.

The problem with going on a raw-food diet without cleansing is this: When the average person goes on raw foods, even for just a few days, the body begins to cleanse. Eating a raw-food diet will not clean out the mucoid layers, but raw foods *will* initiate serious cleansing. What's wrong with that? Well, it brings up cleansing reactions. The average person is so full of toxic waste that a completely raw-food diet, without complete intestinal cleansing, could stir up more problems than most people want to handle. Fruits are the most cleansing of all; vegetables do not cleanse nearly as rapidly. It is ironic that because of cleansing reactions it sometimes appears that eating fresh, raw food makes a person sick, while eating cooked or junk foods makes a person feel temporarily better. All that has really happened in this scenario, however, is that the eating of junk foods has stopped the cleansing process.

Cleansing reactions on a raw-food diet, without cleansing the digestive tract first, can be so severe for the average person that a lack of energy; a "spacey" feeling; eruptions of the skin; and overloads on the kidneys, liver and other organs can be weakening to the point of ineffectiveness. I read of a death actually occurring because the person was exceptionally toxic and ate raw fruit only, for a long period of time. This is, unfortunately, why many who began a raw-food diet eventually concluded that raw foods were bad!

Another factor in the ability to adapt to a raw-food diet is the emotions. Remember, thoughts and feelings are the primal directive force that control our bodies; this includes our appetites and desires. Some people will never be raw-fooders until they have transmuted certain emotions. Thus, I recommend that we *first* cleanse the intestines, then work on deeper levels of cleansing and not radically try to force ourselves to do something that we are presently not ready to do.

Once the digestive system is repaired, you will be strong enough to cleanse the rest of the body. Cleansing should be done gradually and carefully. This is why I occasionally suggest eating a baked potato to those having *extreme* cleansing reactions on any Phase of my program, for this instantaneously slows internal cleansing and they feel better immediately.

Whenever possible, however, I would still prefer that a person suffering those reactions first try an enema.

I spent 20 years trying to cleanse the cell structure of my body first. I fasted a great deal, and although I did not always eat the way I should have between the fasts, I did quite well until an accident kept me from exercising. (Exercise assists in the removal of toxins.) Then it was downhill, with occasional ups during my fasts. Eventually I learned to cleanse the intestinal tract, and my health skyrocketed!

What to Expect as Your Intestinal Tract Becomes Cleaner

One of the problems that occurs when our bodies become more pure is that we begin to notice the effects of the dead foods much more profoundly.

My wife and I decided to experiment with that contrast. After a great deal of intestinal cleansing and a couple of months on raw foods (mostly fruit), we went back to eating the average American diet, minus meat, for four days. Each morning it became more and more difficult to get out of bed, let alone to feel good. We each began to develop the world's worst case of baggy eyes until by the fourth morning we had pouches instead of bags. Wrinkles in the face became decidedly more pronounced. My vision became more and more fuzzy, though by taking my herbal formula for eyes, better sight was restored. Tiny little bumps developed on our skin (as the body made its desperate attempt to eliminate the toxic overload). Our complexions became dull and lifeless. We noticed that our love for each other lessened. Our sleep was interrupted by weird dreams. Our whole bodies became slightly, but noticeably, puffy, and this was especially noticeable in our faces. Our energy levels became lower and lower and, for the first time in years, we found ourselves getting sleepy during the day. I felt some pain in my kidneys, and we both experienced inflammation in various joints. We felt congested in our sinuses and throats as well as various aches and pains throughout the body. My memory became less effective. We both found it difficult to turn our attention to God. Our appetites for food became almost uncontrollable, and we were hungry even when we were still full of food. Work became *work*, instead of the joy it usually is for us. We experienced feelings of low self-esteem and a lack of confidence. We had extended stomachs. Our mental efficiency lessened, and we became more and more prone to negative feelings. We were easily irritated and short-tempered. Our bodies developed foul odors that had been absent for a long time. Being neither TV watchers nor moviegoers, we were amazed when we actually felt the desire for such entertainment.

Believe me, we were so happy to get back on the Cleanse and feel better again, we marveled at our enthusiasm. The bags under our eyes disappeared in three days. We looked bright and felt good again. Our energy returned along with our increasing love and gratitude for each other and for God. In fact, almost every one of the symptoms we had developed disappeared within three days of cleansing.

A few weeks later, we tried the experiment again, eating cooked foods for another four days. This time we even ate chocolates and pizza, but of course we would never eat meat. The same symptoms of ill health and lifelessness returned gradually. It was after this experience that we truly embraced the raw-food diet with the fervor of religious converts. We have developed an appreciation for God's raw, fresh foods that bring joy just in looking at them in their lovely, pure simplicity. Eating God's untampered fresh foods brings greater life and energy into us instead of depleting us. It makes us feel good, our breath is fresher after eating, our mental capacity is increased and uplifted, and our love and joy towards all life is gradually accelerated. Blessed is the life that grows and provides real food, and blessed are those who eat it in its raw and fresh state!

Our earnestness and zeal to conquer all desire for non-foods still remain. We know, so help us God, that all such lower desires will one day be merely fading memories, as we go forward on the path to complete purification.

How to Combat the Effect of the Occasional "Pig-Out"

If you have been working on cleansing yourself, but have the occasional splurge, or "pig-out," as the popular and accurate saying goes, you may experience regrets because of what your body is going to have to go through. You may want to eliminate the effects of the "pig-out" as rapidly as possible. Here is what you can do:

- ❑ Take one serving, plus a little more (if needed) of my herbal Formula 1.
- ❑ Drink extra water.
- ❑ Take one heaping teaspoon of papaya powder .
- ❑ Take as much cayenne as you can stand.
- ❑ Take an enema before bed and one in the morning.
- ❑ Take a psyllium shake when you get up in the morning.

By noon the next day, everything will be okay again. Once, during our four-day experiment, we ate in what appeared to be one of the nicest restaurants in Klamath Falls, Oregon. We had "good ol' " pancakes and omelets, which we hadn't had in ages. The pancakes tasted so bad that I could only eat one of them. A piece of ham, which to me ranks the highest in levels of repulsiveness, was on the omelet; there was also some chili on it, with meat. I picked it out as best I could and ate the egg. Yuk! It was the worst omelet ever. This was the ideal eating experience to help destroy all desire for cooked foods. We laughed all the way through breakfast.

About one-half hour later, I decided it had to go. We stopped the car. I swallowed about four squirts of super-powerful lobelia extract – that's two-and-a-half times the regular dose required to induce vomiting. Then I thought about what I had just eaten and took two more eyedropper shots, undiluted, straight into the mouth. Nothing happened. I couldn't believe it. I repeated the process, using almost half an ounce of the lobelia extract. Believe me, that's enough to make a rhinoceros "upchuck his cookies." Either the lack of reaction I experienced was just plain karma, or else we can assume that the cleaner the body becomes, the less effective lobelia is in its emetic effects. Even though I never did vomit, the lobelia did make me feel enormously better. A half-hour or so later, we both took a psyllium shake, using a whole fluid ounce of hydrated bentonite, and we both felt well the rest of the day.

If there's anything we have learned, it's that it is not beneficial to force yourself to eat any certain way for long periods of time. Give up things gradually, but occasionally force yourself to eat raw foods for at least a few days at a time. Then, without guilt, go back to what you desire. You're going to do this anyway, and it is better to do so without guilt. For, guilt ties us to the very problem we feel guilty about. If you have a strong desire for perfect health, you will eventually lose the desires for non-foods, when your body is ready to let go of them. I do not mean to imply that you should not set goals or give your body a good nudge in the right direction once in a while. But don't impose lofty goals upon yourself and set yourself up for failure and disappointment before you are really ready to embrace your noble effort and take it to the limit. Ask God to help you. If you're persistent without frustration, you'll get there. Read inspiring books about raw-food diets.

Secrets of Super Health

Keep in mind that fruit is the natural food for a clean, healthy body because it has the highest vibratory frequency of all foods. It is this higher vibratory level that allows man to tune into his true nature and his relationship with God. It has been said that God works for man, through man, as man, *when man is pure*. "Only the pure shall see God," warns the Bible. Granted, we must first cleanse and purify our minds, emotions, and actions. Removing the inharmonious feeling from within is more important than cleansing the body. But we cannot do one without doing the other, for the condition of the physical structure affects the mind and emotions, and vice versa. At the risk of being redundant, I will now repeat the following, which explains the state of man and his ability to raise himself. Now, please follow this closely:

- ❑ Our cells, proteins, and mucoid plaque constantly radiate consciousness, just as everything does to some degree; they emit a vibratory frequency which reflects the thoughts and feelings we were experiencing at the time we ingested the protein that became our cells, mucoid plaque, etc.
- ❑ When the mucoid plaque breaks up, memories surface that can exert a significant influence. When the plaque is evacuated it and its inherent consciousness no longer have any effect on us.
- ❑ Therefore, after the mucoid layers are thoroughly removed, it is much easier to eliminate and control desires, appetites, and bad habits as well as negative thoughts and emotions.
- ❑ Cleansing the intestinal tract and eventually our cell structure opens a great potential for peace, harmony, and happiness.
- ❑ Certain foods – those of the highest vibratory level – should be eaten to maintain a purity of mind and body, and foods of a lower vibration (such as meat) should be avoided to shut the door to unwanted vibratory feelings. Eventually all our cells will be capable of eliminating every negative thought, feeling, habit, or attitude once and for all.

My theory is that once we achieve this advanced state of purity, we will have become beings of tremendous love and joy, and true health will be ours. Chances are, the aging process will also be reduced to a snail's pace.

One secret to super health is to so cleanse the entire intestinal tract that one can live an energetic, happy life sustained by raw fruit alone (or Light alone – "breatharians" actually do exist).

Before reaching that point, I believe we will evolve into vegetarians, eating both raw and cooked foods, and then progress to eating a diet of raw fruits and raw vegetables, and then just raw fruits – when we're ready.

Before reaching that state of purity in our diet, all of the above-mentioned foods are appropriate as well as the occasional grains and squashes. Dr. Jensen advocates the use of these four grains only: millet, rye, yellow cornmeal, and brown rice. They should be whole and natural. Sprouted grains and seeds are considered vegetables and provide a tasty source of excellent nutrition, live enzymes and life force. Any foods other than those just mentioned will actually undermine our efforts and lead us backward. However, they can sometimes prove useful when controlling cleansing reactions.

Why Raw Foods are the Perfect Food

Raw foods are the perfect food for man and can bring him exceptional health. They keep the body clean and congestion-free. Only raw foods have life force and enzymes, which are far more important to your health than vitamins, minerals, and amino acids. Vitamins, minerals, and amino acids can keep you alive, but life force and enzymes will keep you *vibrantly* alive. **Foods *with* life force and enzymes *always* offer vitamins, minerals, and proteins as well**, while foods lacking in life force and enzymes at best can only offer minerals, proteins and perhaps some hardy vitamins that may have survived the rigors of whatever food processing methods were used (which destroyed the life force and enzymes.)

Alexis Carrel of the Rockefeller Institute and two-time recipient of the Nobel Prize, **was able to keep tissue cells alive indefinitely** by nutritious feedings and by washing away tissue excretions. The cells grew and thrived as long as evacuations were removed. Unsanitary conditions resulted in lowered vitality, deterioration, and death. **He kept a chicken heart alive for 29 years** until someone failed to cleanse away its excretions!

The same holds true in the human body. If not kept clean inside, congestion occurs, the blood becomes impure, and the result is lowered vitality, dis-ease, and a broken-down immune system, which eventually leads to death. How many times have you marveled at the seemingly endless energy of a young child? Before the body is congested, when it is in its pure state, it is wonderfully alive, vibrant, and bursting with energy. Congestion, which generally begins in the intestines, is really the number-one killer in the world. Without congestion, the cells easily repair themselves. **Dr. Carrel believed that the cell was, therefore, immortal, and he was a very wise man**. Congestion starves the cells of needed nutrients and oxygen. Dr. West, a colleague of Carrel's who has worked in the same field, claims one cannot die without congestion. The body is not only capable of repairing itself, but what's more, it never stops trying! All we have to do is get out of its way. Most people know that putting sugar into the gas tank of a car clogs up the engine, so that the car stops running; eating cooked and processed foods is like putting slime and glue into the body. No wonder the body wears out; it's been forced to work a few too many overtime hours!

So, the key is to eat foods that keep the body congestion-free. And that means raw fruits and raw vegetables. Moses lived 120 years; Methuselah lived over 900 years. Who knows how long *we* may live as we move towards becoming totally pure beings.

Life Force

Life force is the most powerful and effective contributor towards good health that exists. It is the source of energy and nerve power. It gives life to our cells and to the enzymes in our body. It is related to the sun and to breath – both life-essential forces!

Every atom of our bodies is filled with electricity or life force to some degree. These atoms are composed of electrons and protons, which are negatively and positively charged particles. The greater the force, charge, or voltage of each atom, the more power it can generate to feed the life of each cell. The cell itself can be so charged with life force that it can become radiant light. It is this light that repels dis-ease. Light is life. It is energy in its purest form. The greater the power flow, the more one is able to think clearly and accurately. When this energy flows in full force through the nerve channels and emotional body, health is assured and it is easier to maintain positive and loving attitudes. Charismatic qualities of happiness and joy surface more readily. The mind and heart are naturally drawn to higher things. One is inclined to express love and kindness more freely and seldom tires at work or play. And when this life force flows through every cell of the body, we ward off dis-ease, handle stress effectively, stay healthy longer, and ultimately slow down the aging process.

Victor Schauberger (1885-1958), an Austrian naturalist, recognized life force in water. He found that water could essentially die, and could then be restored by interpolating life force back into the water. He recognized that the difference between dead and living water was miraculous. As a hydrologist, he was able to send logs with a higher specific weight than the water down long logging chutes sometimes for miles. The logs "and even stones, floated almost like cork in these specially designed chutes – designed to keep the water vibrantly alive."[125] As long as the water contained the life force, he was able to float huge logs with only inches of water down through the chutes, but when the water was void of life force, the logs would sink and plug up the chutes.

Life force can also be likened to the shields of the *Enterprise* in the *Star Trek* TV show and movies. **When our life force is strong, there is no germ that can enter our inner sanctum.** A healthy body is a vibrant body, and vibrancy is life force.

The life force of the body is not dissipated or destroyed by overexertion (for exercise eliminates toxins, and hard breathing helps draw the life force back in). It is dissipated or destroyed by drugs, dead foods, and negative emotions and attitudes. Each time we consume dead or devitalized foods we are, in effect, "shutting off" our energy, our aliveness, our health, our life force. And the process of aging is increased. A good illustration follows: When one fully-charged 12-volt battery is hooked up to a dead 12-volt battery, the dead battery will draw from the charged battery until the median level is reached. The fully-charged battery becomes considerably drained – in fact, it is drained to half its original force.

And so it goes when eating dead foods. A portion of our life force is automatically drained from our life force reserves to feed the devitalized foods. On the other hand, eating raw foods helps build the life force, adding zest and energy while keeping the body free from congestion. Eating raw food is like eating fully-charged battery cells.

Once we have eliminated all congestion from the body, along with the congestion of negative thoughts and feelings, the life force connection with our Creator and with the solar system may flow in unlimited power through the other centers of the body (which are sealed in most people). Who knows the potential in this? Only those who have attained this exalted state know, and they are the legends in mankind's history. Ponder the well known words of Jesus from the Bible: "All the things I have done you can also do and even greater things shall you do." What do you suppose he meant by that? And what did he mean when he said to his disciples, "Preach ye unto all the world, saying, 'Strive to receive the mysteries of light, and enter into the kingdom of light, for now is the accepted time, and now is the day of salvation."[126]

---

[125] Olof Alexandersson, *Living Water - Viktor Schauberger and the Secrets of Natural Energy,* (Bath, UK: Gateway Books, 1982), pg. 36. Distributed by The Great Tradition, Lower Lake, CA.
[126] S. G. J. Ouseley, ed., *Gospel of the Holy Twelve*, Chapter 65:7 (Pomeroy, WA: Health Research, 1974).

Enzymes and Healthful Eating Habits

Raw foods are full of enzymes. Cooked and processed foods have *none*. Enzymes play a vital role in the digestion of our foods, in fighting dis-ease, and in breaking down foreign matter as well as with almost every metabolic function. With a decrease of enzymes, a process of internal decay rapidly develops, creating mounting problems in the body, which can even be transmitted, through DNA, to one's future children.

Enzymes are essential in maintaining internal cleanliness, not to mention health, youth, and strength. They are far more important than any nutrient: we cannot live without enzymes. Proteins cannot be utilized without enzymes, nor can vitamins and minerals. Enzymes are destroyed after use and must be constantly replaced. Cooked foods draw from the enzyme reserves, depleting the body's precious "labor force." Life force is the central core of each enzyme. Enzymes are the vehicles through which life force works on the physical level. Vitamins, minerals, proteins, and body chemicals all depend on enzymes to fulfill their purposes. Enzymes are the physical activity of life in our bodies.

According to Dr. Edward Howell (who has been considered by many to be the world's authority on enzymes), *each person is given a limited supply of body-enzyme energy at birth.* The faster we use up our enzyme supply, the shorter our life span, the weaker our immune system, and the more quickly our bodies become dis-eased. As he puts it, "The habit of cooking our food and eating it processed with chemicals, along with the use of alcohol, drugs and junk food all use up tremendous quantities of enzymes from our limited supply." He also says that colds, flu, and other sickness deplete the supply.

Dr. Howell exposes the unsuccessful attempts of modern medicine to heal dis-ease and its failure to attack the root of the problem. He says that **many, if not all, degenerative dis-eases from which humans suffer and die are caused by excessive use of enzyme-deficient cooked and processed foods**. This is one of the many reasons that herbs cure and drugs do not. Drugs have no life – no enzymes. But herbs do.

Heating food to more than 116 to 120 degrees destroys all enzymes, and most vitamins, and forces the body to deplete itself. This causes the digestive organs to enlarge, especially the pancreas. Hot foods and hot drinks will injure the enzymes in the stomach.

On a physical level, enzymes are the active ingredients that cure dis-ease; on an *electrical* level, *life force* is the active ingredient that cures dis-ease. Together they comprise the central core of the immune system and are necessary for the maintenance of health and a long life. It is the enzymatic and life force activity that makes your brain function, as well as your memory. It is what keeps your body alive. So, for a longer, healthier, and happier life, one should eat less and eat only raw foods. Whether you believe the following words from *The Essene Gospel of Peace* are the true words of Jesus Christ, matters little, for they offer exceedingly good advice, either way.

"So eat always from the table of God: **the fruits of the trees, the grain and grasses of the field, the milk of beasts, and the honey of bees.** *For everything beyond these is of Satan, and leads by the way of sins and of diseases unto death. But the foods, which you eat from the abundant table of God, give strength and youth to your body, and you will never see dis-ease. For the table of God fed Methuselah of old, and I tell you truly, if you live even as he lived, then will the God of the living give you also long life upon the Earth as was his.*

For I tell you truly, the God of the living is richer than all the rich of the earth, and his abundant table is richer than the richest table of feasting of all the rich upon the earth. **Eat, therefore, all your life at the table of our Earthly Mother, and you will never see want.** *And when you eat at her table,* **eat all things even as they are found on the table of the Earthly Mother.** *Cook not, neither mix all things one with another, lest your bowels become as steaming bogs. For I tell you truly, this is abominable in the eyes of the Lord.*

Take heed, therefore, and defile not with all kinds of abominations the temple of your bodies. **Be content with two or three sorts of food,** *which you will find always upon the table of our Earthly Mother. And desire not to devour all things, which you see around you. For I tell you truly, if you mix together all sorts of food in your body, then the peace of your body will cease, and endless war will rage in you. And it will be blotted out even as homes and kingdoms divided against themselves work their own destruction. For your God is the God of peace, and does never help division. Arouse not, therefore, against you the wrath of God, lest he drive you from his table, and lest you* *be compelled to go to the table of Satan, where the fire of sins, dis-eases, and death will corrupt your body.*

*And when you eat, never eat unto fullness. Flee the temptations of Satan, and listen to the voice of God's angels. For Satan and his power tempt you always to eat more and more. But live by the spirit, and resist the desires of the body. **And your fasting is always pleasing in the eyes of the angels of God.** So give heed to how much you have eaten when your body is sated, **and always eat less by a third.** Let the weight of your daily food be not less than a mina, but mark that it go not beyond two. Then will the angels of God serve you always, and you will never fall into the bondage of Satan and of his dis-eases. Trouble not the work of the angels in your body by eating often. For I tell you truly, **he who eats more than twice in the day does in him the work of Satan.** And the angels of God leave his body, and soon Satan will take possession of it. **Eat only when the sun is highest in the heavens, and again when it is set.** And you will never see dis-ease, for such finds favor in the eyes of the Lord. And if you will that the angels of God rejoice in your body, and that Satan shun you afar, **then sit but once in the day at the table of God.** And then your days will be long upon the earth, for this is pleasing in the eyes of the Lord. Eat always when the table of God is served before you, and eat always of that which you find upon the table of God. For I tell you truly, God knows well what your body needs, and when it needs."*[127]

Friendly Bacteria

"Friendly" intestinal bacteria are essential to good health. Most raw foods, especially those with chlorophyll, feed the friendly bacteria, whereas cooked and processed foods feed the harmful bacteria. The friendly bacteria are needed to:

- ❑ Reduce cholesterol in the blood,
- ❑ Produce certain necessary digestive enzymes,
- ❑ Control the pH factor or acid/alkaline levels in the intestines,
- ❑ Reduce pathogenic bacteria in the intestinal tract,
- ❑ Reduce high blood pressure,

---

[127] Szekely, pg. 41.

- Detoxify poisonous material in the diet,
- Strengthen the immune system,
- Prevent colon irritation, constipation, diarrhea, and acne,
- Manufacture and assimilate B-complex (which includes niacin, biotin, folic acid, riboflavin, and Vitamin B-12,
- Help digest proteins, carbohydrates, and fats,
- Produce natural antibiotics which inhibit 23 known pathogens,
- Produce cancer- or tumor-suppressing compounds,
- Detoxify hazardous chemicals added to foods, such as nitrates,
- Assist calcium assimilation,
- Help eliminate bad breath and gas,
- Prevent yeast infections,
- Help alleviate anxiety and stress,
- Retard proliferation of vaginitis, flu, and herpes.

It's interesting to me that opponents of vegetarianism insist that if one doesn't eat meat, one has no source of Vitamin B-12 and is undernourished. That theory is rather upside down. Those who eat meat destroy the B-12 as soon as they cook it. Also, meat eaters generally have a very poor intestinal flora and are therefore unable to produce or assimilate B-12 properly. Studies have shown that vegetarians who have healthy intestinal flora are able to produce it with no problem at all.

Following is a list of the most dangerous enemies of the friendly bacteria, in order of importance to be avoided:

- Drugs – especially antibiotics, as one dose can eliminate all friendly bacteria. Studies have shown conclusively that those who have used antibiotics have an increased chance of future dis-ease.
- Alcohol – destroys enzymes and bacteria, not to mention actual cells, particularly brain cells.
- Meat – feeds the *Bacillus coli* (harmful bacteria) which in turn destroy the good bacteria (yes, the body is like a living episode of *Star Wars*!).
- Bread – especially white flour, or any wheat bread that was baked in an oven.
- Sugar (processed) – found in most breakfast cereals, chocolate, cakes, pies, cookies, ice-cream, pop, etc.
- Fried foods – e.g. potato chips, French fries, and all fried foods.

Because good health depends on having a balanced intestinal flora, there are many who constantly try to implant the healthy bacteria by taking *Lactobacillus* in its various forms, such as *Lactobacillus acidophilus*. They generally fail in their efforts for one of two reasons: 1) *Lactobacillus acidophilus* will not implant properly in humans, for it is not natural to humans, and 2) *Lactobacillus acidophilus* is highly acid-forming, and the body will attempt to remove it.

Most bacteria formulas (Probiotics) contain a predominance of **acid-producing** bacteria (*Lactobacillus acidophilus* etc.), which are highly beneficial under various pathogenic conditions. However, when used consistently, these bacteria contribute towards abnormal bowel acidity, which is very challenging to the electrolyte balance as well as to a healthy bowel environment. Some studies have shown that patients suffering from metabolic acidosis may have triggered this potential death-causing extreme by consuming *Lactobacillus acidophilus* tablets and/or milk and yogurt containing *acidophilus*. **What are people doing to future metabolic functions when they saturate their bowels with acid-forming bacteria, thereby producing large amounts of unnatural lactic acids consisting of a pH of 3.9 to 4.5?** Doesn't this tend to reverse what the bowel is attempting to accomplish when it secretes fluids of 7.5 to 8.9 pH? And what does this do to the digestive enzymes of the small and large intestine, which **can only function optimally in a pH of 7 or above?** Clinical studies have shown that this has the potential to become a problem of the future, and may have caused death in certain people.

Is there a place for acid-forming bacteria such as *Lactobacillus acidophilus?* As I've said, "Yes, absolutely." In fact, acid-forming bacteria could save a person's life or help eliminate severe disorders. It can also serve to help balance the bowel environment. Some strains of *Lactobacillus acidophilus* create lactase, which may assist lactose-intolerant people. It has been shown to help reduce serum cholesterol and create a wide spectrum antimicrobial activity (antibiotic). Some strains, such as DDS 1[128], have shown anti-carcinogenic activity against particular cancer cells, especially those found in the esophagus, stomach, colon, prostate, breast and pancreas. It has also been shown to modify and inhibit the growth of *Candida albicans*. However, ***Lactobacillus* should not be used as a permanent implant.**

What, then, are the ideal bacteria for man? Studies indicate that *Bifidobacterium infantis* is the predominant species in the feces of breast-fed infants. This is the first bacteria that young, healthy infants receive from breast milk, and may be the most essential and basic bacteria for the human gut. Other *Bifidobacterium*, such as *B. longum,* which are closely related to *B. infantis* and are found in both healthy children and adults, and

---

[128] "DDS 1" refers to the Department of Dairy Science, at the University of Nebraska, where Dr. Khem Shahani developed the products that bear this trademark.

198

Bifidobacterium bifidum, which is found in healthy adults, may be the most natural and essential bacteria for man. Clinical studies have shown that out of all the other *Bifidobacteria* strains tested, both *B. infantis* and *B. breve* were most effective in repelling *E. coli* and *Salmonella,* and their toxins.

These bacteria generate a pH between 6.5 and 7.0, which is much more beneficial for a healthy human bowel than the lactic acid-producing *Lactobacillus.*

And if I *still* have not got your attention here, let me state that beneficial bacteria begin to die off at a pH near 4.5, the pH normally produced by *Lactobacillus acidophilus.* This in itself shows that *L. acidophilus* may actually destroy the beneficial bacteria that are *natural for man.* Therefore, *Bifidobacterium* must be, by far, the dominating bacteria in the gut. *Bifidobacterium* species are also known to produce large amounts of amino acids and other nutritious elements, including vitamins and Vitamin B-12.

Now you know why Nature designed mothers to breast-feed their babies and why children who are *not* breast-fed have significantly more physical and emotional problems.

After cleansing the intestinal tract, implanting the friendly bacteria for the natural healthy intestinal flora, and eating raw foods, you will be well on your way to a healthy, happy life!

CHAPTER 15

TAKE BACK YOUR POWER – RECLAIM THE STRENGTH OF YOUR SOUL

"The survival of every animal, bird, fish, plant, and germ (whether it be bacteria, viruses, fungus, or protozoa), depends entirely upon its environment. Pathogenic germs cannot overcome a clean, healthy, and vibrant human body."

– Rich Anderson, N.D., N.M.D.

Germs are Not the "Cause" of Dis-ease

In my book *UnCreating Dis-ease*, I explain this in depth, but to put it in just a few words, germs – and by that I mean bacteria, yeasts, fungi, molds, parasites, and viruses – **have little or no power over a truly healthy body and mind!** It is only after we have contaminated and weakened our minds and bodies that "germs" have an influence. And we weaken our bodies by what we eat and think. To clarify: **it is what we do to ourselves (diet, lifestyles, emotions, etc.) that develops a specific internal environment in which dis-ease and germs can thrive!** This is one of the most important statements in this book. Forgive my repeating it, but this fact needs to sink in. Please read it again and ponder it carefully. And now, get this! One of the *primary* problems with conventional medicine is that it fails to recognize the following truth: **"Germs" can only live in bodies that are susceptible to the germ**. A vital, healthy body has an incredibly strong defense system. We must weaken our bodies before germs have a chance to live within us. And once we have created that condition, we can also "uncreate" it.

The present medical concepts are devastating to the public, for they fail to address the physiological and psychological factors that allow a germ or dis-ease condition to develop! Remember this and teach your children this truth: **Germs are never the first cause of dis-ease; they are the result of a *series* of SELF-INFLICTED injuries, caused by**

living unnatural lifestyles. It is disobeying the natural laws of life that causes us trouble. In other words, living a life under the influence of ignorance, appetites, and foolish desires is what leads to dis-ease; cancer, heart dis-ease, AIDS and all the other dis-eases of our foolish modern society are *CAUSED* by the *same* series of SELF-INFLICTED injuries. We do not acquire dis-ease, WE CREATE IT! Dis-ease is a natural result of living an *unnatural* lifestyle; it is the breaking of natural law.

Is it worth it? Are all those years of gluttony worth dying a horrible death by cancer? Will the years of boozing it up and eating innocent and helpless beings of Nature be worth spending the last few decades of your life being incapacitated by heart dis-ease, osteoporosis, arthritis, and/or bowel dis-eases? Will the years of gluttony and riotous living be worth having your feet amputated because you created diabetes? Will the years of thoughtless lifestyles be worth many years of suffering constipation, obesity, pain, and bleeding because of colitis and other bowel dis-eases you created? Will the last few decades of observing yourself becoming gradually blind, deaf, and stupid be worth the many years of living a life which was out of balance with Nature?

Perhaps it is time to become strong. Perhaps it is time to look within ourselves and at Nature and discover a new lifestyle that results in vibrant health, strength, joy, and love. It is not easy to undo the many years of mistakes, gluttony, and misuses of the energy of life, but every effort makes us a little bit stronger, and if we persevere, we can "uncreate" our troubles.

Some will ask, "If this theory is true, then what about tiny children who suffer and who haven't had a chance to live a life of gluttony and to misuse Nature's laws?" A good question, and one that each person should have the answer to, but unfortunately, our so-called civilization is so entrenched in such deep-seated *self-ignorance*, prejudice, and beliefs, that the true answer is foreign to them, and they hypnotically evade and ignore it. If the answer is not obvious, then you need to study yourself, and if you follow an intelligent path, the answer will waste no time coming to you. My book *UnCreating Dis-ease* addresses this important subject.

The Power Within

One of the worst crimes of the 20th century is now before you. Our society, and especially those working in medical science and the forces behind that industry, have been willing to exploit a nation, and even a world, for the purpose of control, money, and power. They have succeeded in brainwashing and hypnotizing the vast majority of the "Western World."

This of which I speak is one of the primary causes of such rampant dis-ease, suffering, and limitation in this world today, especially the epidemics of heart dis-ease, cancer, and immune related dis-ease. And if what I said about the influence of germs being relative to our internal environment makes sense to you, then the following should also.

When a person accepts the "germ theory" of modern medicine, **and believes that germs have greater power over their lives than do their own actions, vast, subtle and disastrous repercussions result**. Our nation has accepted the hypnotic concept that we are at the mercy of germs, and many other "things." I am sure that you have noticed the programing activity on television, radio and the newspaper – i.e. how pharmaceutical advertisements talk about "flu season," etc. – which subtly drives their messages deeper and deeper into people's subconscious. They want you to believe that we are at the mercy of germs and that our only salvation is medical drugs, especially vaccines. They want you to believe that you have little power over yourself and that changing your ways is useless. The public has fallen for it, hook, line, and sinker. Millions believe that either they or someone they know will "catch" the flu during the winter, for they have been convinced the programming is true, and they expect its fruition. Unless of course, they have gotten a flu shot.

Seldom do people ask **why some appear immune while others are devastated**. Oh, how in the world did our forefathers and foremothers ever survive for the many thousands of years without the intervention of modern medicine's vaccines and drugs? And **why is there more chronic and degenerative dis-ease in this world than at any other time in our history**?

It hardly ever occurs to people in present times that they have any power over themselves, let alone over germs. **People have been literally bred to deny their own innate power to control their own being!** Therefore, they are now at the mercy of the modern medicine – that is, if they have the money. And so it is that when a doctor tells patients that they will die, 99% of the time they will die, **for they believe in the doctor more than in their own innate ability to take charge of their lives and health!** People have lost their power! No, that is not quite true; **people have unconsciously given their power to those who will misuse it and will make money from it at their own expense!**

Most people of our society have become just like the cattle that are bred for slaughter! The consumer has become the consumed. The manipulators do not eat us like people eat cattle, but **they feed off the weakness and stupidity of mankind, like parasites**. Over 99% of our society dies from **unnatural** dis-eases. And for only one reason: **people**

have failed to intelligently use their own innate power, the power given to us by our Creator. And this has happened because of our education and programming. One of the main reasons that people have fallen for this fraudulent conspiracy is simply that their **minds have become dulled, so subtly and unconsciously dulled that they are unaware of their dull state, and unaware that they are being manipulated.**

CHAPTER 16

THE EXPERIENCE IN TEESHI LUMBO

"When Magellan sailed around the tip of South America, he came to a certain island, anchored his ship, and with some of his men, rowed to shore. They were met by natives and were able to communicate with them. The natives were astounded, and wondered how they had come to the island. The Captain pointed to the huge ships in the bay and said, 'We sailed here in those great ships.' The natives, who had good eyesight, looked long and hard, but were unable to see the ships. Were those ships so far beyond the experience and comprehension of the natives, that their ability to see and believe was blocked?"

– Dr. Rich Anderson

North Cascades

In August, 1987, White Crow and I hiked about eight miles over a high mountain pass into Teeshi Lumbo Valley of the North Cascades in the state of Washington. Truly this is one of the most magnificent, secluded, and rugged mountain valleys in the continental United States. First we had to wade across the rushing Chiwawa River. Then we hiked up an old dilapidated trail, which winds up through steep, rugged brush, forests, and rocks until it breaks into high, mountain meadows that stretch for miles on end. The first day we hiked until dark, which brought us past some rocky cliffs at the base of a meadow developed by annual avalanches, where the year before we had seen a bear and her cub. Then we broke into the high mountain meadows, which were filled with heather and blueberries. It was here that we ate our last peaches, nectarines, and *acidophilus* (a big mistake). This was to be our last meal for six days, for our purpose was to fast in this mountain wilderness, drinking only fresh, living water.

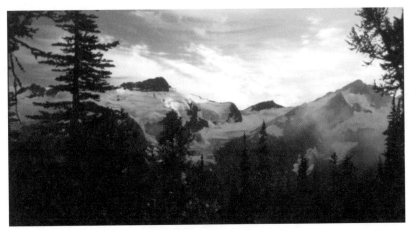

High Mountain Pass

The next morning we hiked up over the pass and down into one of the most scenic mountain valleys on Earth. By the time we descended to the valley floor and reached the river, we were already feeling the full effects of the fast, for we had been living on raw fruits with occasional salads for several months and our wise bodies had already initiated a deep cleansing activity. We had just covered many rugged miles of exceptionally steep terrain, carrying full backpacks, since we intended to stay as long as three weeks. The hot sweat rolled down our bodies, and the combination of such a clean diet, strenuous exercise, and now the water fast put us into a maximum-cleansing mode.

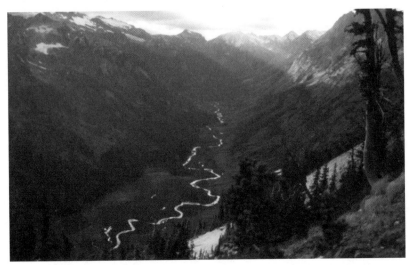

The Valley

205

As we set up our tent, we were feeling tired and weak, partly because of the fast and the exercise, and partly because of the acidophilus.[129] We then took a plunge into the icy cold of the glacier-fed river and washed off the sweat and dust. This helped us regain our strength. White Crow, more than any other person, had fully convinced me of the therapeutic advantages of cold water, how it could bring strength and healing. We had taken hundreds of icy cold plunges together, and I was quite impressed with what Mother Nature can do for us through cold water. This river was indeed cold, as its source was only a few miles upstream and was fed by mighty glaciers. The water was, in fact, glacier-silt water. It was so clouded with silt that we couldn't even see our hands when submerged just inches below the surface. This plunge truly had marvelous effects on us, and we immediately felt much better.

The sun had already descended behind the glacier-speckled domain, for the mountain range ascended steeply almost 5,000 feet above us. With the sunset, the temperature dropped quickly and the air, being crisp and clean, also had a sharp bite to our wet and bare skin. We were many miles from any road, so there were no other people, no noise, and no pollution or any sign of it. This was how we began that memorable water fast.

Three days passed, and we were both feeling worse on this fast than on any other fast or cleanse we'd ever undertaken. But thank God for the cold rushing river; truly we were saved by our cold baths. We sincerely yearned to be rid of all toxins, poisons, the dark emotions, and anything else that interferes with our connection with the Great Spirit. The cleaner, the more pure we became, the more immaculate we aspired to be. We had developed a driving compulsion to become totally pure and to have the rare privilege of associating with those who have reached the ultimate purity – those who became "like angels in Heaven." Not only had we been working on purifying the physical body, but we had been striving to purify every thought, feeling, appetite, desire, and even belief. We strived to eliminate all selfishness and egotism from our beings, for we recognized that a lack of humility was an automatic rejection of the great Oneness. The moment anyone thinks of himself or herself as special or unique, that person

---

[129] Usually on a water fast, we would begin feeling good after three or four days. That is why we were willing to go so far into the mountains and fast; we were confident in this fact. However, as an experiment, we took large amounts of acidophilus at the beginning of the fast. We continued to think that we would be feeling better any day, but this didn't happen. It wasn't until several years later that I finally realized that the acidophilus was creating extraordinary acids that contributed to most of our weakness during that fast. Through the combination of excessive exercise, lack of food, and the acid-forming bacteria, we had drained ourselves of electrolytes.

unconsciously acknowledges a separation from Oneness – the Great Spirit – God. Our experiences had vividly proved to us that this was a serious mistake, which, by the grace of God, would be overcome. We strove to be as little children – without the contamination of foolish opinions and judgments – as clean mirrors that easily reflected the Son. Much progress had been made, and we still had a long way to go, but we hoped that this water fast in the exceptional purity of this mountain environment would speed our progress. And so it was; even beyond our expectations.

Angel of Light

It was the evening of the third day and the sun had set hours before. Though I was tired, I was also compelled to finish reading the book *The Gospel of Peace of Jesus Christ,* by the Disciple John.[130] Crow was already fast asleep, and I had to use a flashlight to complete the last few words of this highly inspiring and informative booklet. I was deeply touched and inspired by its wise words and I wondered, did it really happen that way? Were those truly the words of Jesus himself? I wished fervently to know. Then I crawled into my sleeping bag, hoping that we would sleep until noon of the next day, for our bodies were so weak that it was almost unbearable to crawl out of our tent to our no-walled bathroom.

As I was uncomfortably lying there, my thoughts turned to Barbara, my wife (at that time). I let my thoughts drift with her. I soon entered the magic place – that place between sleeping and waking – and I just let my imagination wander deeper and deeper into an enchanting Devachan. We were walking through beautiful, landscaped gardens, up a walkway to a pure, columnar, white temple. Appropriately, we were both dressed in pure white. We were preparing to enter the temple when an elderly couple, also dressed in pure white, approached. I recognized them. They had recently used my cleansing program. Their faces glowed with health, a light shining in their eyes revealed their gratitude for the benefits derived from their cleansing experience. As I looked upon their beaming faces, my love went forth with great intensity. I went up to them and put my arms around them both and unconsciously uttered these words:

---

[130] This booklet contains the "pure, original words of Jesus, translated directly from the Aramaic tongue spoken by Jesus and his beloved disciple John, who alone among Jesus' disciples noted with perfect accuracy his Master's personal teachings." It is part of a manuscript that exists in Aramaic in the library of the Vatican and in old Slavonic in the Royal Library of the Habsburgs (now the property of the Austrian government). This volumn is also known as *The Essene Gospel of Peace.* For more information, see the Bibliography, under Szekely, the editor and translator.

"Blessed art ye, for your willingness to purify yourselves." I was filled with a tremendous sense of appreciation for their willingness and efforts to purify themselves.

Tears of joy and love welled up in my eyes and then increased, until I felt embarrassed at my overflowing gratitude for their strength. I turned to Barbara and wrapped my arm around her shoulder. Then an unexpected wave of love with unusual intensity flooded over me. We walked to the trees and my love and appreciation for her increased in exponential, cyclic waves, until I awoke from ecstatic thrills of love never before experienced.

I lay there for a moment stunned by this extraordinary bliss. At first I thought I had just had a wonderful and powerful dream. But then another wave of even more intensity flooded through me so powerfully that I realized that I was having another ardent Divine experience. I could feel an intense vibration all through my body. I lightly placed my fingers upon my arm to see if I could my feel skin vibrating. I attempted to comprehend this powerful and unusual pulsation flowing in me. Then, somewhat disappointedly, I realized that my body was simply too impure to handle this much energy much longer. I sensed that if this vibration continued for a few hours, my body would begin to disintegrate – it simply was too weak, too impure, to handle such a potent charge. But, I did not care if my body disintegrated; if that meant I could continue being in the presence of this much love, then let it be so! I had no fear of death, none whatsoever. As I bathed in this immeasurable love and happiness, tears of gratitude and pure joy continued to stream from my eyes, dampening my sleeping bag. I just wanted to continue feeling this Divine bliss forever.

Suddenly, another even more potent wave of love shook my body, and with it came the most loving, sweet words: **"Blessed art thou for thy willingness to purify thyself; thou shalt be rewarded openly, if thee will persevere!"**[131] My eyes flew wide open, and to my utter joy and astonishment I saw right through the tent, where directly above it hovered a massive, brilliant, and star-like, white light. I intuitively knew, from the core of my being, that I was in the presence of She whom the great Master had spoken of in the *Gospel of Peace of Jesus Christ*: the Earthly Mother. Words cannot describe Her. She was surrounded by an aura of light so bright that I could see only brilliant light that was scintillating. Instantly I had the desire to see into this light, to see the form of its source. I struggled to see, and slowly Her form grew more and more vivid. She had long,

---

[131] It would be more than a decade later before I more fully understood what was meant by "if you persevere." At that time, and for several years later, I had no idea just how tough it would be. Many times I was close to giving up, but instead, I continued to persevere.

golden hair, which fell below her shoulders in waves, and large, bright eyes filled with energizing and potent love, infinite wisdom, knowing, and compassion. Her Presence was extremely potent, yet the feeling was calm and peaceful and I felt perfectly at ease, as though I were a young child in the arms of my mother. I could clearly see the awesome energy and power radiating from her – indeed, her eyes shone like the eyes of Christ. No mortal's eyes could compare. She floated just a few feet above the tent. Millions of tiny, quarter-inch light rays rippled in various colors – blue, gold, pink, green, violet, purple, aqua, and white – flowing gently, but intensely, in all directions from the sphere of Her being. I studied those wonderful light rays, trying to absorb and learn everything I could. Truly, I did not wish to miss a thing.

I knew that She knew every single thing there was to know about me, and that far exceeded what I knew about myself. I felt no embarrassment for my weaknesses and impurity, for I was being embraced with a source of true love and compassion. Suddenly I was filled with new and vast information, which, a few seconds before, had not been within my awareness. With absolute certainty I understood her message, at least to the degree of my understanding and experience at the time. She explained to me that anyone and everyone who willingly purified themselves and sought love – not only physically, but also mentally, emotionally, spiritually, completely, and persistently – would receive rewards beyond their fondest dreams. For it is through purification that we can become vehicles of immense love and intelligence, and it is the impurities that contradict and block the Infinite love and intelligence. And it is only through complete purification that we can truly know our real self – the Higher Self, which is the Christ connection with the Oneness of all life. Mankind has no idea as to the power of love and what it can do. With enough love, there is no poverty, no sickness, no death, and no limitation, except for what we consciously choose. The presence of enough love solves every problem, every hurt, every limitation, and all lack. All happiness is a product of love, and the more love, the greater the happiness. Enough love dissolves selfishness, greed, hate, fear, limitations, and struggle. The more we love, the more the Infinite Oneness flows though us, for God is Love.

I then understood the biblical words, "Only the pure shall see God," and I yearned for that kind of purity. My desire was – and is – intense and sincere. I also realized that purification is a necessary ingredient for entrance into what is called Heaven, and that only those may enter therein who have first been purified. The human ego, the part of us that wallows in selfishness, vanity, lust, anger, and fear, and views itself as separate from the vast Oneness that is God, enters not, for it is in direct opposition to Oneness. And those who postpone their purification will return to this earthly life over and over until they achieve the destined purity. I also learned that those who desire the greater purification shall have the assistance of God's mightiest messengers and, if necessary, legions of angelic beings. I see that the ultimate purification is the ultimate destiny of human evolution. This must be accomplished before one is conquered by the last enemy: death.[132] For, after death, little progress is made, and one must come back and try again.

Even though this knowledge has been available for thousands of years, and was emphasized by Jesus Christ, only a few seem to grasp its significance. Only a few have been strong enough to make use of it, for as I said, it is in direct conflict with man's lusts, appetites, and desires. Divine Love offers divine benefits, while man's lusts, desires, and appetites offer only temporal pleasure, well-mixed with pain and suffering. I have also learned that Love and joy are the natural antidotes that relieve the limitation associated with pain, fear, and suffering. As light dispels darkness, so do Love and joy dispel suffering. When Love and joy are expressed, there is no consciousness of suffering.

I have now realized that the greatest gift we can ever have is to love others and that we should love our so-called enemies, if for no other reason but the pure joy of loving. And as light dispels darkness, so also does purity dispel evil and suffering, and purity is unconditional love for everyone and everything.

I listened to Her words and was then allowed to ask questions. My first question was, "Were the words written by the disciple John in the *Gospel of Peace of Jesus Christ* the actual words of Jesus?" Her answer: "With the exception of a few translation errors, those words are the words of Jesus, and are true."

About then, I strongly desired that White Crow see and experience this; though I found it difficult to move, I managed to jab him in the back with my elbow. He awoke and rolled over. I found that I couldn't talk, and he rolled back over on his side. I jabbed him harder – oops, a little too hard – right on his backbone. He turned over and said, "Rich! Why did you do that?" I struggled to talk, and finally managed to utter the words: "Crow, look above the tent!" He uttered a cry of astonishment, for he also clearly saw Her wondrous presence and felt her endless love and compassion. It is always more enjoyable to share these experiences with another. For about 30 minutes we talked, and for those 30 minutes, we were filled with an essence of such love that it made all things on Earth seem small and insignificant in comparison.

---

[132] Jesus said, "Verily, verily, I say unto you, if a man keep my saying, he shall never see death." John 8:51.

When our conversation was nearly complete, She asked me to include this experience in the next publication of my book. A fear arose that this would inhibit sales of the book. I struggled with it for a moment, and then replied that I would do so. Then She said that She would come again. She kept her promise and gave me another invaluable lesson – a lesson that eliminated every excuse not to love all life everywhere, no matter the circumstances. She then began to arise and shine. She ascended straight up and, as She did, She grew in size and brilliancy. The higher She rose, the larger and brighter She became. By the time She reached the top of the mountain's multiple peaks, She seemed to be over 500 feet tall. Strangely, Her pure, white light formed a golden radiance, which lit up the entire valley almost as though it were day.

There are those who walk physically on Earth and yet live in a "Heaven on Earth." They are masters of themselves, because they conquered the human ego of selfishness and all its contaminants. They have become individualized focal points of the Oneness of all life – Love. They all teach that it is not the "i" – the little i (the human ego) – that accomplishes this exalted state of Love, but rather the Higher Self – that part of our inner nature which knows its Oneness with Christ. True freedom is obtained only at the point where the human ego lets go. The crucifixion is but a symbol in which man's ego dies, and then the Divine, or Christ, takes full control. My angel friend was once like you and me, but through purification of Her Being, she became One with the One Life, the One Love.

It is my hope that regardless of people's religious beliefs, that they will be encouraged by these words to strive for truth, love, and purity. I have attempted to show that it does not pay to create inharmonious thoughts and feelings, and that the only sensible use of our energy is to love. Each time we remove a dark thought or feeling, we are a little closer to greater love, better health, and to achieving our greater potential.

After this astounding encounter, three days went by, and it was the sixth day of our fast, when we awoke and I felt that a shift had occurred. It no longer felt right to continue fasting. I expressed my feeling to my white-bird friend, and he expressed his feelings too: "Rich, I wanted to quit on the second day and you talked me out of it. Now I want to keep going with this. I'm not stopping."

"Crow," I said, "it isn't that I want to break the fast. We have gone through the worst part and the best is just ahead, but something deep inside tells me that we must stop for reasons I do not understand. Let's go take a bath and maybe we can get some answer on this." We crawled into the icy

211

river, floated downstream, hiked back up and repeated the plunge again until we were so cold our bodies began to turn blue; but our energy increased and we could think more clearly. Then we waded out to the island, sat on the sand just where the water met from both sides of the island, and there we meditated and received our answer.

So, we hiked out the next day with great difficulty. It was a very steep climb, and in some places the slope was almost vertical. When we were about three-quarters of the way up the mountain, we stopped to rest. Crow took off his pack and balanced it upright on the edge of the trail; it was sitting in a rather precarious position. We plopped into a patch of wild currants and blueberries. Our appetites were screaming. Suddenly, Crow's pack tilted and began to roll down the mountain. I thought, "Oh no, it will take hours to get it back, and neither one of us has the energy." Crow quickly stood up and commanded his pack to stop. The slope was about a 60-degree angle, but to my absolute surprise, it stopped.

In obedience to the request of Her who came to me, and in the hopes that this story would indeed assist and encourage others, I did place this in my book. As anticipated, I was criticized and received many letters from people who accused me of talking to Satan, and who were convinced that I must be evil. But I also received many letters from grateful individuals whose intuition told them the story was true. They shared that this story gave them encouragement when they most needed it.

So, what did this experience do for me? Thirteen years have passed since it occurred. If you are one who is aware of Jesus' teaching that "By their fruits ye shall know them," perhaps you would like to know: Did this experience produce positive or negative effects?

The experience gave me encouragement to aspire towards greater purification, and it produced an insatiable desire to love others and also to stop judging, and to accept others as they are. This has not been easy for me, for I had a great deal of stored up anger and resentment; and the more I had seen the depths of the corruption and dishonesty in this world, the more I was tempted to become even angrier. But this experience gave me the desire to never quit working to overcome my failings. When I was tempted, and I certainly have been tempted, I persevered. I found that I was pained each time I hurt another, even though it was slight and deserved. Although I had always felt a desire to help others, that desire increased and expanded until it included the whole world. I have felt a steady increase in my desire to be a pure instrument of Divine Love and also to associate with those who are "like angels in heaven." I am much less selfish and strive to function with the very highest integrity and honesty. For I have realized that whatever we do unto another, we essentially do unto ourselves, and to all life, even to those great and wonderful Christ-beings with whom I yearn to associate with every fiber of my being – I would rather die than lose that opportunity. So I have dedicated my life and energy to assist life everywhere I can; to help our angel friends in bringing love and peace to this world, and to do it without force or violence, but only with love and awareness. And in pursuing this purpose, I have found more and more happiness and love flowing through me; that is what this book is really all about.

And to those who have read this, who believe it, who are encouraged by it, and who seek that ultimate purity, I would like to say, though we may not have met, you are my brother, or sister. We are friends and more, and I pray that you will also be rewarded along your path with experiences of love such as this story records.

CHAPTER 17

TROUBLE SHOOTING:
QUESTIONS AND ANSWERS

This Chapter is devoted to answering the many questions that people have asked over the years.

Q - I was on my second day of the Master Phase of the Cleanse and followed the directions to the letter. I felt pain in my lower stomach. It continued to get worse and by the third day I had to stop the Cleanse, for the nausea and pain had become unbearable. I had passed a lot of the mucoid fecal matter, so I know that it is in there. I want to keep cleansing. What should I do?

A - You did the right thing by stopping the Cleanse. Having seen the iris of your eyes and knowing what you just went through, I would say you may have some serious parasite activity. You're fortunate to have discovered it at such a young age. I am actually a little surprised, because your eyes indicated that you are far above average in your health, in your overall constitution, and internal body cleanliness. You have no history of colitis or stomach problems. You followed the directions perfectly and had good elimination. Many people who had pain and nausea while on the Cleanse suspected parasite infestation. Each of these people who stopped the Cleanse and followed my Parasite program never had a problem with either pain or nausea after going back on the Cleanse again.

Q - Do you recommend using digestive aids when I'm not on this cleanse program?

A - Yes, if you feel that you need them, and usually that will be until one is eating only raw foods and has cleansed and strengthened the digestive system. Remember this: Proteins and carbohydrates require different sets of enzymes. It is best to take enzymes specifically designed for amino acids and another set for carbohydrates. Green papaya is one of the best completely natural sources of enzymes that works for both types of food, and many people swear by it. Green papaya powder not only helps heal the digestive tract, but also helps dissolve undigested protein in the gut. (Since undigested proteins are the number-one favorite food of parasites and pathogenic bacteria, getting rid of them takes a tremendous burden off the body. However, the body also uses protein to coat heavy metals for safe storage. Thus, in cases where heavy metal toxicity may be present, *intensive* intake of enzymes must be avoided, for it could trigger the release of heavy metals into the system. A person with heavy metals should limit enzyme use to only what the body needs to digest current food as it is eaten. If heavy metals are an issue, I suggest using my very effective heavy metals program. Contact my office for the most current information.)

Green Papaya Powder contains a complex of enzymes that help digest proteins, fats, and carbohydrates. It's loaded with Vitamin A, C, E and B factors. It is the highest source of papain you'll find, which is a superior aid to pepsin and pancreatin. It is good sprinkled over food (especially salads). You can feel it harmonizing the body.

Q - Does it cause any problems to keep liquidified trace minerals and bentonite in plastic containers?
A - Storing the minerals in a food-grade plastic is not a problem. However, it is possible that bentonite could leach particles out of the plastic. I recommend that when keeping bentonite for a long period of time, you either keep it refrigerated, or purchase it in a glass container.

Q - What do you recommend for P.M.S?
A - Cleanse, eat pure foods, and use high-quality herbal extracts. Make certain that you have plenty of electrolytes. Take both organic electrolyte and trace mineral supplements for at least 30 days, and a full spectrum of antioxidants just before you would expect P.M.S to appear. Be sure to avoid constipation, especially during the few days before and during menstruation. Stay away from salt, meat, dairy, sugar, and wheat products.

Q - I take that "psyllium shake" and my stomach hurts!
A - In all the years I've been helping people cleanse, I have known this to happen only six times. Two people were taking too much psyllium, two had worms, and the remaining two were White Crow and myself. Here's what happened to us: After reaching a state of health beyond anything I'd ever experienced before, we were on our way to the North Cascades. It was 2:00 A.M. when we reached Eugene, Oregon. We needed some rest. Since we prefer the stars to motels, we slept outdoors about 200 yards from a sheriffs' training area. Just at the crack of dawn, helicopters began flying low, passing right over us. They continued for a couple of hours. We assumed they were practicing training maneuvers. As we were about to leave, a woman came over to our car and warned us that we had probably been sprayed with the "Gypsy Moth BT" chemical. Bless her heart! She gave us some information concerning the spray, and we looked for signs such as residue on the car or our sleeping bags, and we sniffed for chemical smells. We found nothing, and we felt fine. However, about 24 hours later our stomachs had swollen beyond anything we had ever experienced before; we began burping a horrible chemical stench, and then

began uncontrollable vomiting; we felt terribly disoriented; we lost our coordination; we had uncontrollable appetites for heavy acid-forming food; we became mentally incapacitated; and to top it off, we later developed rashes which turned into oozing, uncontrollably itching welts. We were unbelievably miserable! We stayed at my mother's in Seattle for one week, lying on our stomachs night and day. After vomiting everything out of our stomachs, we could only upchuck small amounts of white, chemical foam. Finally, I realized that all I needed to do was take some bentonite in water. Within a few minutes, the vomiting stopped and I immediately began to feel better. Then we headed for the mountains to try and heal. Using bentonite, I was able to rid myself of the rash in less than a week. For some reason, Crow refused to use the bentonite and his rash lasted over a month; and it was three (3) more weeks before his stomach bloating and burping stopped. But then we were feeling much better, and after completing our herb hunts, we headed back to Mt. Shasta.

One night on our way home, just south of Salem, we camped in a vacant lot. It was late. We didn't think that "BT" sprays would be there because we were in a different county. And it had been almost a month since they had sprayed in the other county. However, just 24 hours later, it happened all over again – bloated stomachs, vomiting, and this time diarrhea. Crow had it even worse – he had slept on the grass; I had slept on a tarp.

We parked the car at the ski bowl on Mt. Shasta and hiked about one mile to our camp and fasted, for we were unable to eat. About then, my toenails turned black and one of my front teeth also turned black, and after a few weeks it became brittle and broke. After two days of lying on our stomachs, Crow convinced me to try eating baked potatoes. We drove to town and bought some potatoes and had a feast. This treatment failed, and we became worse. It was dark when we left the car and slowly hiked up to our bare camp spot; we had no tent. It took me about an hour, for I had to stop and vomit three times, and experienced severe diarrhea three times. When I finally arrived at the camp, I could barely climb into my sleeping bag, and I lay there for about 36 hours. Why didn't I think to use bentonite?

After a few days the body stored away the sprays it was unable to release and we improved to the point that we could at least function somewhat normally. About a month later, I finally went on the Cleanse, which is what we should have done in the first place. I began to have pains in my stomach. Why? Because my body began to release the sprays it had conscientiously stored in a cyst-like case. It wouldn't let those chemicals go through my system and destroy itself. The body demonstrates fantastic intelligence! Then the psyllium-bentonite shake began to extract the "BT" sprays. I immediately felt better, so I increased the bentonite. POW! I was in pain! Because the pain was so great, I stayed flat on my stomach once again, but only for one night.

Each time I vomited I smelled those chemicals. Finally, I vomited a cyst of white, slimy mucus and – bingo! – it was over for good. I soon felt good again and my mental abilities returned. I shook my head in disbelief that I had been so mentally incapacitated that it took me so long to realize the solution. It was several months later when White Crow finally used the Cleanse, and he had exactly the same experience. After passing a "huge, white, slimy fuzz ball," as he called it, he immediately felt better and his normal strength and ability returned. No more stomach pains!

> Note: The "Gypsy Moth BT" spray is said to be nontoxic to humans; believe it or not! This pesticide is said to kill gypsy moths by destroying their digestive system. Well, it almost destroyed our digestive systems, and had we gone to a medical doctor, I am certain that we would still be having problems. Fortunately, we knew something about natural healing and we used Mother Nature's natural ingredients, which eliminated the cause. The spraying of toxic chemicals on public lands is a crime against life and against our Mother Nature. Think about how many animals must suffer horribly from pesticides and herbicides. If ever you have the opportunity to give your input at public hearings about this issue, I would urge you to do so.

Q - Will I lose much weight during the intestinal cleanse?
A - Obese people often lose a great deal of unwanted weight while on the Program. I know one man who lost 68 pounds while on the Cleanse, and he still had more he wanted to lose, but he was very pleased. Thin people usually lose very little weight and usually gain whatever they lose about two or three days after finishing the Cleanse (minus the weight of whatever mucoid layers they passed). Sometimes thin people will continue to put on weight after cleansing because their digestion has improved.

Those who cleanse do not lose muscle, only fat and mucus. The only exception might be with those who are suffering from heavy-metal poisoning or who have a life-threatening dis-ease such as cancer. And of course these people must cleanse more than anyone else, but they have to do it with great care and take special supplements.

Q - Is it okay to take a colema or colonic?
A - Yes, absolutely, especially colonics. They are highly recommended, even over enemas.

Q - Can the enema water flow into the small intestine?

A - Only if your ileocecal valve is somehow stuck open. But that is a rare malfunction. There are two causes for this: mucoid plaque blocking the valve from closing, and a nervous reflex condition that blocks the message for the valve to close. If you suspect the latter, call a naturopathic doctor, who should be able to help you. Massage may also do the job.

Q - Will the intestinal cleansing remove diverticula?

A - I believe that it can – eventually, and as long as proper eating habits, exercise, enemas, and herbs are consistently utilized.

Q - I don't want to take enemas anymore. They make me feel weak.

A - I have seen this happen several times. Again, it's because of the toxins. One or two enemas are simply not enough. I suggest a colonic or a series of enemas. Flush out those toxins! I knew a man who suffered terribly from hypersensitive environmental illness. When he took enemas, he would just fall apart, which wasn't very far from his normal experience. I tried over and over to get him to take more enemas, but he refused. Finally, about a year later, he took five (5) gallons of enemas, and by the end of the day he felt the best he had felt in many years. Knowing the difference at that point, he plunged deeper into cleansing, and overcame his problems, which allowed him then to live a normal life.

Q - Should I continue to take my medication while on the Cleanse?

A - I really cannot advise you on that one. I am not a "drug doctor." It can be dangerous to suddenly discontinue their use. Even though most drug doctors have no experience with cleansing, I must advise you to discuss this with your drug doctor. As a rule, the more you cleanse and the more pure your diet, the greater an impact any drug, herb, or food will have upon your body. For an example, diabetics almost always gradually cut down on their insulin while cleansing. Most of them use only half their normal amount after they complete just one Cleanse.

Vegetarians, who live on a clean diet, cannot handle the normal dosages of drugs. Doctors need to learn this! I have seen vegetarians go into shock with a normal drug dosage. I know of one case where a routine drug was given to a vegetarian woman who had simply become dehydrated during her pregnancy. The drug caused her to go into shock, and a few days later she died. Remember, medical drugs killed close to 400,000 Americans in 1996, and the number increases each year. As I said, very few drug doctors, M.D.s, understand cleansing or vegetarian diet. They will almost always prescribe way too much, and it almost always injures people. Our bodies were never meant to partake of these *unnatural* chemical drugs. A true doctor should use herbs, and rarely drugs. A true doctor would be in alignment with nature – not against nature! Those who really know natural healing know that, in most cases, herbs and natural remedies can replace the need for almost any drug. It just takes more effort and planning, but the person will be far better off in the short and long run if he uses natural healing. Never forget, 99% of medical doctors do not understand natural healing – cleansing, herbs, vegetarianism, or anything else I've discussed in this book. Even the medical doctors who write books about herbs, etc. are very ignorant of what true natural healing is all about. There may be some, but I am only aware of one. Not only that, I do not find very many naturopaths whom I believe qualify as true naturopathic healers. They're too ingrained in the medical propaganda, and these days even what is taught in most naturopathic colleges parallels medical concepts.

Q - I have a weak heart. I notice that during this Cleanse it pounds a lot.

A - I used to have a weak heart too. In fact, I'm also supposed to have bad valves and an enlarged heart because of having rheumatic fever as a child. My heart used to pound and skip beats occasionally while cleansing. Releasing drugs and other toxins can make anyone's heart do that. But it doesn't happen to me anymore. If you are truly concerned, take cayenne pepper and hawthorn berry. No drug can strengthen the heart like these two herbs do. Cayenne, especially in a tincture, can stop a heart attack or stroke in less than 30 seconds.

Your question reminds me of my mother, who is one of the "neatest" people you could ever meet; she gets straight A's in personality. She had always trusted the AMA's treat-the-symptom syndrome. Her faith in that arena has now dwindled to a low ebb, but only after watching her mother die a horrible, unnecessary, slow, painful death, and after having seen so many of her friends and relatives suffer needlessly. Until then she had always marveled at the wonders of medical science. When her hip started giving her trouble, she began to hope for a bionic hip. I did my best to try and convince her to try healing herself Nature's way – with herbs. My efforts were in vain. She eventually received her wish and now has a bionic hip. She loved it! But after her operation, she never seemed to enjoy her original active condition, and her heart was actually causing her serious problems. She kept taking all of the wizard-like concoctions her doctor would give her, but to no avail – he simply did not know how to repair her heart condition. Finally, one day I left her just a few cayenne capsules saying, "Mother, it can't hurt you! It's just food. There's nothing better for your heart! Just take two and see what happens." She said, "Well, maybe," as I left.

The next day she was exhausted once again. She was just going to take a mid-morning nap on the couch. She went into the kitchen for one more coffee and saw those cayenne capsules lying on the counter and decided to try one (even though I had told her to take two). She swallowed it down, went upstairs to the bathroom, searched for a book to read, and headed for the couch. She started to lie down and suddenly stopped and said to herself: "Wait a minute! I'm feeling pretty good!" Not only did she dispense with the nap, but she ended up spending the whole day working in the yard, and called to tell me to order her a large bottle of cayenne. Since that one (1) cayenne capsule (she was 78 at this time), she continued taking the cayenne along with hawthorn and never had a single sign of a heart condition for several years. Cayenne is loaded with Vitamins A and C, and potassium – the heart mineral.

Q - I'm pregnant and would like to start cleansing. Is it okay?

A - No. Though many pregnant women have successfully used the Cleanse with great success, there are certain risks. Ideally, every woman should cleanse her body temple before becoming pregnant and then be sure to acquire the best nutrition for herself and her new baby. In America, each generation has become weaker and weaker because of drugs; vaccines; chemicals in air, water, and food; and mainly because of poor diet. The toxins that can arise during a cleanse could affect the fetus. They can also affect mother's milk after the baby is born. My suggestion for the potential mother is to drink at least one or two cups of red raspberry tea each day during pregnancy, and to eat an organically grown alkaline-forming diet. Drinking this tea can solve many problems and make the entire pregnancy and delivery easy, enjoyable, and successful. Each woman must seek the advice from within and make her own decision as to how to conduct her life.

Q - I've been told by my doctor that I have a spastic colon and that I'd better be careful with colon cleansing. What do you think?

A - I agree. Be careful. If I had your condition, I would cut down on the recommended dosages of psyllium. I would also use catnip-tea enemas made with distilled water to relax the colon; I would be very generous with the amount of catnip. Believe me, though, if I had a spastic colon, I sure wouldn't hesitate to cleanse. I would do anything and everything I could to repair that area now and not wait until I became worse.

Q - What about using bentonite in my enemas?

A - Not recommended except in extreme cases such as severe colonic infections of *Entamoeba histolytica* – the protozoan parasites that kill so many people who have AIDS. That would certainly knock them for a loop. Even though clay, especially bentonite, is an excellent healer, it is also highly caustic to the epithelium wall and can actually injure this delicate membrane.

Q - Is it true that friendly bacteria can be destroyed when you take a colonic?

A - It washes them out. But chances are, if you need a colonic, you need friendly bacteria too. I *always* take my probiotic formula each time I take an enema.

Q - My menstrual periods have changed since I've been cleansing. Is that normal?

A - Actually, that is common among women who cleanse. Menstrual cycles often change as the body becomes purer. Contrary to popular belief, bloody menstrual discharges are not natural to pure women. The purer a woman's body becomes, the less discharge there will be, until eventually there will only be a minor mucus discharge. I had a friend who, after one-and-a-half years on raw food, followed by two-and-a-half years on fresh fruit only, found that she no longer had any menstrual discharge. People used to guess her to be 23 to 29 years old and never older – she was 44! Few women ever get to this level, but it is common for women who have massive discharges before cleansing to find that after each cleanse, the discharge decreases. This is especially true if they eat a raw-food diet between cleanses.

Q - If I eat yogurt, do I still need additional bacteria?

A - Yes. First of all, the bacteria in yogurt is usually acidophilus, which is not recommended for replenishing bowel bacteria, and there isn't very much of it in a serving of yogurt. But think abut this: Why, after going to all the trouble of cleansing would you want to recontaminate your body with the mucus and congestion that accompany dairy products. Truly it is counterproductive. One exception: if the yogurt was freshly made, from raw goat's milk, it would probably be very good for you.

Q - I've noticed that there are other psyllium products on the market that contain added enzymes, herbs, bentonite, and acidophilus, all in one container. Wouldn't that be a better way to go?

A - The herbs, enzymes, and bacteria must be taken separately from the psyllium and bentonite for a definite reason. The action of psyllium and bentonite is to attract and bind elements and carry them out through the body. The herbs must be free to mix with the mucoid plaque so that they can condition the plaque to break off from the gut wall. Enzymes do nothing to mucoid plaque. And once the bacteria touch bentonite, the bentonite will either dehydrate and destroy them or bind them and carry them out of the body. So you see, any enzymes, herbs, or friendly bacteria in the bulk mixtures can never be released to do their job. Therefore, the substances in these mixtures are excellent by themselves, but ineffective when mixed together and taken all at once. Not only that, but these mixtures dilute the pulling power of the psyllium and bentonite.

Q - Can I take montmorillonite instead of bentonite?
A - Montmorillonite is the active ingredient in bentonite. In other words, they are the same thing.

Q - Is it okay for my children to go on the Cleanse?
A - You bet! Get them off to a great start. Why make them go through what most of us went through? Children from five to ten years of age should have their dosages of bentonite and psyllium cut in half. Adjust the herbs, too.

Q - Will this Cleanse program work if I continue to eat meat?
A - Yes, but take periodic pH tests. Watch your electrolytes and cleanse more often, because you will recontaminate yourself sooner.

Q - In the past, I've taken medicine, with terrible side effects. Occasionally, I re-experience these side effects when I least expect them. Will cleansing help this?
A - Drugs can settle anywhere in the body, including the intestines. They are like time bombs. Sometime and somewhere, they may come loose from the body's binding elements and enter circulation. I believe that many elderly people die prematurely and/or acquire a dis-ease such as cancer or AIDS because stored drugs and other chemicals, such as heavy metals, reentered circulation after being safely stored for many years. This is likely to occur after a person becomes too weak and has lost too much weight to deal with them.

It would be a wise choice, therefore, to use intestinal cleansing as early in life as possible. In other words, it's better to do this when a person is around 30 years old rather waiting until 90 years have passed. For, although the Cleanse ingredients absorb much of the dangerous substance and minimize its destructive potential, the Cleanse can still provide a significant challenge, especially to someone who is older, more toxic and weaker. Though elderly people have achieved wonderful results with cleansing, they may need to be more careful than most younger persons.

Q - Will the Cleanse help the immune system?
A - The body's natural immune system cannot be repaired in a toxic body. If your body is toxic, it is already overworked, stressed, and weak. To rebuild the immune system, internal cleansing is a must. Also, use the following herbs: capsicum, ginseng, reishi mushroom, and astragalus. Notice that I did not include echinacea? We use echinacea to kick-start the

immune system. Never take echinacea for longer than 10 days, for the body builds a tolerance to Echinacea, and then when you really need it, it will have less effect. Keeping the body clean, strengthening the liver, and using the herbs listed above will strengthen the immune system. Diet is also essential, as are positive attitudes and visualizing yourself in vibrant health, which should always be followed by acting "as if" you *are* in vibrant health, even if you must pretend. This sends a powerful and beneficial message to the subconscious. This process is an expression of the powerful spiritual law that whatever is held unwaveringly in consciousness tends to manifest in body and affairs.

Q - Do you recommend the Cleanse for all dis-eases?

A - WARNING: Those with tuberculosis, cancer, emphysema, and diabetes should seek the assistance of expert health professionals who have a high success rate with those conditions. Diabetics should consider fasting only after receiving expert advice to do so. These are all "filth dis-eases," but one must be very careful while removing the filth. Each person has unique conditions and should be monitored by someone well qualified to assist with these specialized applications of the cleansing process.

But, to answer your question, if I were suffering from one of those dis-eases, I would most certainly cleanse. How do you think people get those dis-eases in the first place?

Q - I've heard skin brushing is a good way to cleanse. Do you agree?

A - Absolutely! Soap will not clean your skin as well as skin brushing with a natural dry bristle brush will. (Avoid nylon brushes). Soap removes only a small portion of the dead skin, while skin brushing removes much more of the dead skin and dirt with it. Soap often clogs the skin's pores and inhibits its elimination. Skin brushing stimulates the skin and lymph by causing circulation. Don't let your skin become lazy and overworked when just three minutes of skin brushing before your bath or shower will renew and strengthen it.

Q - *Irradiated foods* – I've been hearing about them and they sound scary to me. Do you know anything about this?

A - Irradiation is a new, tremendously effective and diabolical method of preserving fresh fruits and vegetables that has recently gained nationwide acceptance. It is extremely popular with the supermarkets because it will increase their profits, since their produce will have a longer "shelf life."

Why is irradiation so bad? For one thing, it destroys the enzymes in the food. They put the food on pallets and drive them into huge vaults;

then they seal the door and turn on the *nuclear radiation*. If a person were in the vault during this process, he would die instantly. All this just to make the fruits and vegetables last longer! The reason they do last longer is because there is nothing left alive in them that could cause further ripening. Thus, even when individuals try to eat live foods (and purchase raw, irradiated produce), they are acutally consuming dead foods! It isn't the same as cooked food – it's worse!

Though it is claimed that there are no harmful effects from consuming nuclear irradiated food, no one has ever made the proper tests to determine if that's true. I believe that it is another clever design to help, in the future, to reduce the health of people – thereby further increasing revenue, and eventually helping to depopulate the planet. There is plenty of evidence to support this. The American Medical Association and its partners, the FDA and the drug companies, have gone the extra mile to make America the sickest nation in the world, especially with degenerative dis-eases.

But the good thing about all this is that you don't have to be a part of it. Support your local health food stores, which are trying to provide you with good, wholesome, natural foods. Buy organically grown produce only! Even though it is more expensive, it usually tastes better and has up to 300 times more nutrition than commercially grown produce. Who knows what all those chemicals in and on the supermarket food will do to our bodies over long periods of time? ...or to our children and their children? The FDA is forced to remove toxic chemicals from the market many times every year because it is discovered that something they had previously put their stamp of approval on was indeed very harmful. But then they turn around and allow another new, harmful chemical to take its place, etc. The same thing takes place in relation to drugs.

Constant replacement of harmful drugs with "new drugs" occurs almost daily. How many times have you heard your doctor say, "We have a new drug we're experimenting with." The only reason they are not using the last experimental drug is because either it didn't work or it was found to be harmful. So, now they are trying a new one . . .on whom? Back in 1910, Adolf Just wrote a book called *Return to Nature*. His success brought thousands of so-called incurables to him. Concerning remedies, he wrote the following:

> *"All remedies that have not been taken from Nature, and are not in accordance with her, prove futile; no matter how often they may have operated (seemingly) beneficially and effectively. There are too many deceptions here. The injury that inevitably accompanies all unnatural remedies, sooner*

or later, always comes to the surface and causes them to disappear again, unfortunately only after much harm has been done. Such unnatural remedies come and go, therefore, and will never find an abiding place of refuge.

"We see accordingly new remedies rising to the surface daily in medicine, only to disappear again as quickly as they came. Today carbolic acid, tomorrow palicylic acid, now antifebin, again Koch's lymph is the elixir upon which the safety and happiness of mankind is said to depend, until it has become clear that they work only harm and disaster. At present we calmly allow ourselves to be most seriously injured by remedies whose dangerous character can reveal itself only in the future."

Sound familiar?

Q - Everyone in my family has died of cancer, and I have it, too. Doctors couldn't help them and they haven't helped me. I know that if I'm going to get well, I have to find another way. Can you help me?

A - I would love to help you and I believe I could, but it's against the law for me to do so; I dare not even give you my suggestions, for I live in the state of California in the good ol' USA. Here, as in most states, it is against the law for naturopathic doctors to practice medicine. It's also against the law for those who know how to cure cancer to use their effective protocols. But those who have a success rate of less than 19%, including nonfatal cancers, can treat cancer with methods that have proven to be ineffective and dangerous. Those methods have never eliminated the *cause* of cancer and yet no other method is allowed. Doesn't that just boggle the mind? Do you realize what power the AMA, FDA, and Pharmaceutical companies wield? Do you realize what is behind these organizations? I wish everyone would read *World Without Cancer, Confessions of a Medical Heretic,* and the other publications I've listed in the "Recommended Reading" section at the back of this book.

But of course, how does anyone know that I, and others of my philosophy, can successfully treat anything? Many people I know who have had success in treating cancer had to do so under cover. And each time they get involved, they take a major risk of going to prison. For, in California it has been against the law to treat cancer by any method other than surgery, drugs and/or radiation. They've broadened that limitation a little, but not much. Even the European and Canadian cancer treatments that have proven to be highly effective are still against the law in the United States.

Fortunately, you still have the freedom to do to yourself whatever you want. Watch for my new book; *UnCreating Dis-ease,* which focuses specifically on cancer. Hopefully, it will shock many people into awakening on these points.

CHAPTER 18

TESTIMONIALS

The following are true reports from people who used my Cleansing program.

I'm Pregnant!!!!! – "My health has generally been good; however two years ago I was diagnosed with endometriosis and told I would not conceive. Doctors started me taking a 9-month course of birth control to be followed by Danocryn, which I refused. Symptoms worsened, so I turned to holistic treatments with herbs and magnets. Shortly after that, I was introduced to your Program by Charles B. I completed it last March with great success. My whole life changed for the better. Since then I have continued to cleanse and to eat raw foods. The great news is that yesterday I found out I'm pregnant! I have had no morning sickness. I truly believe I got pregnant because I cleaned out a lot of old toxins that were preventing me from carrying a baby in a safe environment. I feel so blessed to have done the Cleanse. I feel it's the greatest gift I have ever given myself.

I have a health and beauty aids business (for seven (7) years now) with approximately 600 "regular" female clients. I want to promote the Cleanse to all of them. My closest friends are already convinced of the benefits, and six (6) of them are ready to begin the program… As far as benefits of the Cleanse, to name a few…I have more energy than I know what to do with. I wake up clearheaded, don't need coffee, I do skin brushing instead. I'm not sleepy after meals. I feel light and energized. I watch very little TV because I can't sit still that long. Our grocery bill is less than half of what it was before. I'm making everything fresh so I don't concern myself about preservatives. I feel satisfied at each meal because I'm a conscious eater now. I don't snack because I don't have cravings. I feel healthier because my food is moving through me at a faster pace. And I feel younger, which is terrific!"   – Christine D., Spring Valley, California.

> **Warning**: We have four testimonies from women who were told that they could never become pregnant and after the Cleanse became so.

Immune System Restored – "I am now 23 years old, and for the past eight years I have suffered from a total immune system breakdown,

227

beginning with ulcerative colitis, and heightening to relapsing poly-choncritis, which is the immune system attacking and eating away cartilage in the body. Other symptomatic problems I experienced include severe body itching, terrible facial acne, liver and digestion dysfunction, hair loss, low energy level... All "Western" medical philosophies dictated that I would have to endure this for the rest of my entire life; I refused to accept that.

The past eight years of mental battles, vegetarianism, acupuncture, and soul searching have resulted in about 80% recovery. Recently, Marie M. gave me a copy of *Cleanse & Purify Thyself*. After reading it, I realized why all of my health problems occurred in the first place. Years of McDonald's, Jack in the Box, and other poisonous foods of that sort, along with continual year-round doses of antibiotics, had devitalized my digestion, assimilation, and evacuation – thus decimating my body.

"I immediately started on a cleanse – a two-week Gentle Phase followed by one week on the Master Phase. During the Gentle Phase, all my colitis symptoms (constant bloody diarrhea evacuation), which had been gone for so long, returned: healing crisis. During the first three days of the fast, I felt very sluggish and nauseated. On the fourth day my energy level shot up to the level it was as a child; my nose started growing back where the cartilage had been lost; and my itching stopped. Performing two colemas a day during the fast, I evacuated at least 15 feet of black, ropy, impacted fecal matter, shaped like the colon and intestines.

"For the past three years, I have scratched myself, especially my legs, bloody almost every single night! Since my cleanse, I have not itched one single time! My energy is increasing every day and I love it... I now see that no matter how much you take care of yourself, you cannot achieve total health unless your body is clean and pure." – Sincerely, Chad M., Santa Monica, California.

Recovered From The Deadly Effects of Medical Radiation – One health practitioner told about one of her clients, "...who had bladder cancer three or so years ago and they overdosed her radiation treatment, and she had no control over her bowels. They said it'd be that way for the rest of her life. After one week on the Cleanse her bowels are moving on their own in the morning with no uncontrollable diarrhea." – Catherine, Tucson, Arizona.

Bone Cancer Pain Reduced – A man in terrible pain from bone cancer came to me. After his first Cleanse, he reported, "Rich, at least 75% of the pain just disappeared."

Bliss Consciousness – "I'm a 26-year-old male attorney who works very long hours, endures a lot of stress and confronts a lot of unhappiness in both my clients and the courtroom. I used the 10-day Master Phase program and released approximately 18 ft. of hard, stale-smelling fecal matter. Some of my stuff was even black!! I reached a point during the program where I actually felt transcendental – my spirit was freed!!! The 'terrible problems' I faced on a daily basis weren't so terrible, my chronic fatigue disappeared; the bags under my eyes vanished along with the tiny crows feet around my eyes; my handwriting even changed!!! I felt incredible feelings of love for family and friends. I entered a state of bliss that I had never experienced or have not since experienced. I actually felt close to God. Tears come to my eyes as I describe this to you. You must all know that this program is a godsend. Its effects are real and revealing. – Scott B, Port Angeles, Washington.

Critically High Blood Pressure Back To Normal – One woman in California reported to me after she did the Cleanse, "Prior to cleansing, I had very dangerous high blood pressure for over a year. Nothing the doctors did ever helped my condition, but on the sixth day of the Cleanse, I went back to the doctor for a checkup. He was shocked to discover my blood pressure was normal." – L.J.

What Goes In Doesn't Always Come Out – A woman in Idaho reported that ever since she could remember, she had a hard lump in her abdomen. About half-way through the Cleanse she had a very strange sensation just below her stomach. She drove home as fast as she could and soon passed a hard piece of material about six (6) or seven (7) inches long and about two inches thick. She cleaned it off and after her husband looked at it, he hit it on the toilet, and it sounded almost like metal. Then he hit it hard and broke it. Inside were multi-colors. When she saw that, she instantly knew that it was from all the crayons that she had eaten when she was about five years old. From then on, the hard lump was gone. She was so impressed with the Cleanse that she convinced perhaps 50 or more people that she knew to take the Cleanse.

Crippled Woman Walks Normally Again - "For the last seven years, I have been dealing with a steadily increasing amount of pain in my right hip. For the last six months, the pain had become so great that I was using a cane regularly when outside of the house. X-rays showed that the cartilage had worn off the head of the femur. An infection had also developed. The nerves at the head of the femur were telling my brain to immobilize the right leg. In spite of many different types of therapy to reverse the steady downward spiral, nothing seemed to turn the gradual decline around. The different therapies I tried included…chiropractic treatments, therapeutic massage, nutrition, exercise… homeopathy, yoga, as well as colon cleansing using Dr. Jensen's program... Approximately ten weeks ago, I started using Dr. Anderson's Cleanse. I did everything suggested in the book *Cleanse & Purify Thyself.* On the second day of the Cleanse, approximately 50% of the pain left my body and I stopped using the cane at that time. On the third day of the Cleanse, I did a little yoga with my yoga students for the first time in over a year. They were watching me with their mouths open, because their most recent experience of me was seeing a person move with great agony and pain." – Marie M.

Children Benefit Too – A mother wrote, "My six-year-old, after two weeks of the Gentle Phase and mostly raw foods, passed a six-inch chunk of old, blackish-brown, dried mucoid matter with striations... Proof that, 'Yup! He did need it too.' We're both more excited now that we're seeing results. We'll be back in touch post-cleanse... Glad you're there. Thanks." – Pamela

A Woman From Canada Wrote – "I tried it. On the second day I could not believe how good I felt and the stuff that came out of me looked like the gunk when an alien starts disintegrating." – Mrs. D. Urgwhart

Serious Headaches Vanish – "I have had the most excruciating headaches anyone would ever have for many years now. Do you think that you can help me"? I could see that her elimination systems were far from normal and her body was accumulating toxic debris. Soon she was on the Gentle Phase, and after 10 days, went on the Master Phase. She began to lose some unnecessary weight, and before the Cleanse was over she told me the headaches were, for the first time in years, completely gone. She became vibrant and outgoing and started to enjoy life in a way that had been impossible for her up to that time.

First Pain-Free Menstrual Cycle – "...Benefit from first Cleanse: Had the first pain-free menstrual cycle I have ever had in the last 15 years..." – S. A., Hinsdale, Illinois

Back Pain Gone! – "The pain in my back was so severe that I could not lift weights, nor could I walk without pain. Just after my first cleanse a piece of mucoid plaque that was at least 1 1/2 inches thick and over 3 feet long came out of me. It was so hard that I couldn't cut it with a perforated knife. The pain disappeared immediately and I felt stronger, more alert, and from then on I had much more energy." – Ron Sherr, Arizona

Miscellaneous Common Results – "...increased energy, improved circulation, weight loss, clearer thinking, relief from constipation & gas..." – B. S., Alberta, Canada

Cancer – A Pharmacist Wrote – "In Testimony to Rich Anderson's Cleanse of 1991: I received the following benefits: 1. The GID (Gastrointestinal disorder) I had suffered from for years, GONE. 2. The IBS (Irritable Bowel Syndrome), GONE. 3. An Esophageal Reflex condition that was increasing in intensity the past year, GONE. 4. Toxemia of the body, I had developed from above, GONE. 5. Brought to my awareness the mental depression I was in. 6. Changed my eating, lifestyle, and food preparation. 7. Lost 30 pounds. 8. Slowed (reduced) the progress of Prostate Cancer. (23%) 9. Made me develop a personal CHOICE in how I wanted to live my life; physically, emotionally, mentally, and spiritually. I would recommend this program to anyone who has similar conditions."

Joint Pain Disappearing – "...the quality of your products so much surpasses what's out there. They seem like different substances...Pain in joints nearly gone..." – S. B., Los Angeles, California

Cancer; Pain Gone – Plus Happy Side Benefits – "I have lymphoma cancer under my right arm. Talk about pain! After the Cleanse, the pain was completely gone." He went on the Cleanse nine times and lost 75 pounds of unnecessary weight. His overall energy increased two to three times; and he eliminated an enormous amount of "emotional stuff, day-to-day worries, and other basic fears." – Tony Miles, San Francisco, California

A Man In His Eighties – "I was on the Master Phase of the Cleanse for the full seven days. Forty-five feet of beautiful Mucoid Sheaths were expelled. What should I do with it? It is lying on the bathroom floor on aluminum wrap – the answer? I'll take pictures of it. I feel so much better and have more energy to continue my artwork. This was a great birthday gift. I plan to continue experimenting with this. I think that possibly the cataract might be corrected in time." – Alfred Israel, Phoenix, Arizona.

A Mother Wrote Concerning Her Daughter – "I am writing you about your wonderful *Cleanse & Purify Thyself* book and how much you helped my daughter. She was in PAIN for years. It was so bad that sometimes she couldn't speak! She went to doctor after doctor and hospital after hospital and they tested her in all their ways, but couldn't find the reason for the pain. Until she went on your program. Thank you for writing such a brilliant book and helping my daughter lose all that prehistoric fecal matter. She is a new girl. I am going on the program myself." – Romona

Breast Lumps Disappear – "...Almost too numerous to list! A large cyst, very painful, had been growing in one of my breasts for seven (7) years; it dissolved by the end of my first seven days on the Master Phase. Painful, swollen areas of my colon got unblocked. Four inches vanished from my waistline. Lower back doesn't hurt as much. On the 5th day of the Master Phase, lots of goopy, strange (chemical odor) green stuff came out at 1:30 A.M. My menstrual periods are now perfectly in time with the New Moon and not as painful. I have less tension in my upper back, between my shoulders. I'll keep on cleansing until I'm totally renewed..." – P. D., Flagstaff, Arizona

Worms, Parasites, and Crawly Things – "I'm gaining more and more energy, vitality, and have a newfound energy. The total length of worms that came out of me in seven days equaled 335.4 inches." (27.9 feet) – Barney Davis, Tucson, Arizona

Sinus Problems – "Dear Rich: I am writing to encourage you to keep up the great work you are doing. I have used your products and think they are the best. I have suffered for years from sinus problems and virtually all of my troubles were cleared up after my first cleanse. I am more alert, alive and energetic." – Robert Cronin

Diabetes – "Dear Mr. Anderson, when my doctor told me I had diabetes I was really frightened. I had gone to see him because I had no energy. I was always tired and had to stay in bed most of the time. I'm 71 years old and had always had a lot of energy and stamina, so when all of a sudden I had to stay in bed and could hardly get through the day when I worked, I was really scared. My late husband and sister had diabetes and other health problems, and I saw what the insulin and other drugs did to them. It was horrible. My husband and sister had high blood pressure and so did I. My daughter saw you on television and bought your book and had gone on your detox program. She said she couldn't believe how nice her skin looked. She had a terrible acne problem at 48 because of prescription drugs she had been taking. I had prayed and asked God to show me a way out of taking drugs for my health problems. When my daughter told me about your program, I didn't hesitate starting right away. The first week I started on the program I felt an immediate difference. I felt wonderful for the first time in months. I had no symptoms and my energy returned within the first two weeks. My tongue did turn very black about the third week. White Crow said not to worry, my body was just releasing toxins. My tongue turned its normal color after a few days and I have not taken anything my doctor prescribed since I started on the Gentle Phase. Thank you very much, you were the answer to my prayer." – Sincerely, Clara Perea, Tucson, Arizona

Stomach Pains and Lumps Gone – "God Bless You. I love you and I thank you for your Cleanse. Several years ago, the doctors thought I had a tumor and I had to have several ultrasounds. There wasn't one. They sure did not know what was the matter. I had a large, hard stomach and suffered pain a lot. I told one doctor, 'If you can't help me, find someone who can!' During the Cleanse my stomach started to disappear. I was amazed. The hard lumps were getting smaller. I also was constipated, had sensitivity to plants and foods, had floaters, anemia, and edema. Noise pollution had me shaking. I had a flaky rash between my eyebrows and on my forehead in two spots. The rash on my forehead and brow went away just taking the Chompers and my face felt softer within a few days. I used to think that going to the restroom once a day was great, but I realized I was wrong. I started to have three to five (3-5) bowel movements a day with Chomper alone. During the 7-day Cleanse I got 50-3/4 feet out. All my symptoms and pain were gone." – Mildred, Pasadena, California

It Really Works! – "...I found the program to be everything it claimed to be. After years of listening to exaggerated claims and health hype, I have become reserved in my endorsement of products in the natural-healing arena...How very refreshing to find a health system that works!..." – R. D., Arcadia, California

Professionally Endorsed - "I am a colon hydrotherapist who has been involved personally with health pursuits for nearly 10 years because of my own body. I have used Dr. Anderson's program several times and put dozens of my clients on the program. I believe in cleansing and feel the program to be the best on the market for this type of cleanse..." - L. H., Venice, California

Blood Pressure and Heart Rate – "...I was able to stabilize blood pressure & heart rate within first five days of cleansing." – J. H., Pasadena, California

Most Effective Program – "...I have been doing various forms of cleansing for 15 years. Your seems to be the most effective one that I have found yet." – A. M., Penryn, CA

Tumor Decreased – "...I was on the cleansing fast for six weeks and Marjorie did it for five weeks. During that time the tumor (on my left shoulder) decreased in size by about two thirds, my body felt lighter and more pliable than at any other time in my adult years (I am now 65), and I am convinced that the cleansing was in large part responsible for how I feel. I have lost about 25 pounds and intend to continue the fast as recommended in the book." – E. M., Roswell, New Mexico

All Symptoms Gone! – "...Almost all of my symptoms have disappeared. I threw out a shoe box full of prescriptions, and am able to exercise (I can actually take a deep breath, and breathe through my nose. I haven't been able to do that for twenty years!). Oh, my allergies are gone too (dust, mold, yeast, pine and grass pollens, etc.). The cystic acne went away, my weight dropped, dizziness is gone, and heart palpitations are also gone. Prior to the Cleanse I could not grow fingernails. They would break, chip, were thin and would bend and tear. For the first time in 15 years I have long fingernails, all strong, all unbroken and all due to the Cleanse. (I recognize that I am absorbing calcium properly now.) I now have to cut them so I can do some of the things I couldn't do before I took the Cleanse (Oh, poor me! Women pay so much to get nails glued onto their fingers...I have to laugh at myself, now I want to cut them off to learn Kung Fu). I still have some sinus, I feel after my next cleanse more of the prescription drugs stored in my body will depart and more of the 'dreaded mucoid plaque,' ending the sinus symptoms as well..." – P. M., Castro Valley, California

Many Benefits – "...Benefits I experienced include: more energy, better concentration, fewer colds, elimination of a life-long sinus problem, no more menstrual cramps, no more headaches, I sleep better, I have regular eliminations, no more stomachaches, clearer complexion, I look younger, I lost weight, my eyes are brighter, I'm less stressed, etc. etc. etc." – C. O., Los Angeles, California

Never Hungry, Lost Weight, More Energy – "...We both did four weeks on the Gentle Phase. (My husband was a meat eater and a heavy dairy-eater). Then we did seven days on the Master Phase. Throughout the Cleanse, we both worked full-time and we were NEVER hungry!!...My husband had not had a regular bowel movement for 30 years! After completing the Cleanse, he now has two to three bowel movements a day!! After completing the "Chomper cleanse," we both experienced a significant increase in energy. The quality of sleep has improved tremendously. My husband lost 21 lbs. of fat! I did not lose any weight, but dropped two sizes in clothes..." – B. V., Lemon Grove, California

Lots of Plaque – "...I passed about 35 feet of hardened mucoid plaque. I did not feel weak or hungry..."
– P. V., San Diego, CA

Good-bye Hay Fever and Pain, Hello New Lustrous Skin – "This note is to thank you – for your love, compassion, caring, hard work, and research. Your Cleanse was unbelievable! The best thing I've done for myself! 35 feet of 'filthy stuff' came out of me! So many positive and amazing things happened to me! The first real noticeable thing is my skin. It's clearer and has a luster I don't remember it ever having before. Others have commented on it too! I've been seeing an acupuncturist for five months – trying to open channels enough to release excessive amounts of toxins from my body. I've had a large lump in my knee and it's been very painful. But...now... after my first Cleanse, the toxins are all cleared. My knee is great! In fact all my energy is flowing so perfectly now that I don't need to go back to see him for a long while! Yah! (He was very amazed too!) And my hay fever? During the Gentle Phase it started to lessen and during the Master Phase, I had NO hay fever at all. It's now been a week since the eighth day and the sneezing is starting again. I know after a few more cleanses it will be gone for good. I have no words to adequately describe how I feel right now. It's a 'clean' and a 'lightness' I don't remember having. Every time I released more 'stuff' I felt such a relief and love for myself. I guess for me that's the most wonderful thing...a new discovery of love for myself. So... I say please keep working and sharing. I send you all my love and aloha and strength. Much love," – Jennett.

The Average Testimony

People report much more energy, feeling closer to God, feeling better, pains disappearing, the appearance of skin improving, lumps disappearing, mental faculties becoming sharper, eyesight improving, various problems disappearing, obese people losing weight, having better control over the emotions, and feeling happier.

APPENDICES

Appendix I
ALKALINE- AND ACID-FORMING FOODS

Alkaline-forming Foods

All fresh and raw fruits, vegetables, and sprouts, including those listed here:	Grapefruits
	Grapes
	Green Beans
	Green lima beans
	Green peas
Alfalfa sprouts	Green soy beans
Apple cider vinegar	Herbal teas
Barley	Honey, raw
Apples	Kale
Appreciation	Kelp
Apricots	Leaf lettuce
Avocados	Leeche nuts
Bananas	Lemons
Beets & greens	Limes
Berries	Love
Blackberries	Mangoes
Broccoli	Maple syrup
Brussels sprouts	Melons (all)
Cabbage	Millet*
Cantaloupe	Molasses*
Carrots	Mushrooms
Cauliflower	Mustard greens
Celery	Okra
Cherries	Onions
Collard greens	Oranges
Cucumbers	Parsley
Dates	Parsnips
Dulse	Peaches
Figs	Pears
Fresh corn	Peppers
Fresh, raw juice	Pineapple
Fun	Plums & prunes
Goat whey	Potatoes*

Acid-forming Foods

Alcohol
All processed foods
Anger
Barley
Bread, baked
Cake
Canned fruits and veggies
Cereals (all)
Chickpeas
Chocolate
Cigarettes
Coffee
Complaining
Cooked grains (except
  millet and quinoa)
Corn, dried
Cornstarch
Dairy products
Drugs
Eggs
Foods cooked with oils
Fruits, glazed or sulfured
Ketchup
Legumes
Lentils
Meat, fish, birds, shellfish
Mustard, prepared
Nuts, seeds, beans
Oatmeal
Pasta
Pepper, black
Popcorn
Salt

Alkaline-forming Foods	Acid-forming Foods
Quinoa*	Soda crackers
Radishes	Soft drinks
Raisins	Soy products
Raspberries	Stress
Raw, cold-pressed,	Sugar, white and
organic olive and	processed
flax seed oils	Sweeteners, artificial
Rhubarb	Tea, black
Rutabagas	Vegetables, overcooked
Sauerkraut	Vinegar, distilled
Spinach	Vitamin C
Squash	Wheat, all forms
Turnip Greens	
Tomatoes, ripe	
Watercress	
Yams	

*Foods marked with an asterisk (*) significantly slow the Cleanse process, and can reduce the amount of plaque removed. It is suggested that, while on the Mildest or Gentle Phases, the foods with an asterisk be limited to two to three servings per week.

Note: All foods become acid when sugar is added.

How to Make a Vegetable Broth

Take three (3) quarts of distilled water and add three (3) medium to large whole potatoes, two to three (2-3) stalks of cut celery, and one or two (1-2) large leaves of any greens, such as collard, mustard, kale, or turnip or a half-bunch of parsley. Even carrot or beet tops will do. Whatever is green. You can even add kelp if you want high concentrates of a wide variety of minerals. Use a stainless steel pot and bring to a light boil with the lid on. Simmer for 15 minutes. Remove from the heat, and after it has cooled a bit, strain and throw out the chunks, keeping only the juice. Refrigerate. Drink two to three (2-3) cups/day.

VACCINE COMPENSATION LAW

Pressure from parents who had experienced death and disability of their children from vaccines caused Congress to adopt the *National Childhood Vaccination Compensation Law,* authorizing payment of damages to children harmed by immunization. However, Congress failed to convey this knowledge to the public, and apparently, to doctors who administer vaccines. A few years later, drug cartel lobbies pressured Congress to drop this program.[133] However, according to the National Vaccine Information Center, a person can receive federal compensation of up to $250,000 for a *vaccine-associated death,* and may be compensated for all past and future unreimbursed medical expenses up to $250,000. Apparently $250,000 is what Congress thinks a child is worth.

Obviously, this "Act of 1986" was developed not for injured parties, but to prevent the injured survivors from suing vaccine manufacturers and their providers. (See http://shot.com/compen.htm and http://www4.law.cornell.edu/uscode/unfamed/42/300aa-11.html)

But what about the tens of thousands of only slightly injured children? Those who will have health and mental problems for the rest of their lives, but can't prove that the cause was vaccines?

---

[133] Many people consider the vaccination of children the worst crime in the history of mankind. Vaccines are one of the primary causes of the explosion of dis-ease in the Western World. Vaccines are unnatural toxic filth, and it has recently been discovered that they cause the immune system to mutate into impotency. No one knows how many people have died from vaccines, but the figure is undoubtedly in the millions. There is a great deal of controversy about vaccines, yet those who do the research are convinced beyond a shadow of a doubt that vaccines are far, far more harmful that the dis-eases they purportedly eliminate. In the opinion of many doctors, scientists, and researchers, the medical propaganda about vaccines is mostly unscientific and in many cases fraudulent. There is no doubt that many thousands of children, as well as adults, are being permanently harmed, and oftentimes killed, by vaccines. It is a fact, that this is far more common than people think. Those who wish to investigate before they receive another injection, can read some of the books about this subject listed at the back of this book. Take away the profit made from vaccines, and vaccines would disappear. Vaccines are not beneficial, except perhaps in a few instances; they do, however, benefit those who make and sell them.

RECOMMENDED READING

For additional and late-breaking information see Dr. Anderson's web site (http://www.cleanse.net)

Other Books by Dr. Rich Anderson

Available through Christobe Publishing, P.O. Box 1320, Mt. Shasta, CA 96067, (530) 926-8855.

Cleanse & Purify Thyself, Book 2 – More than 340 pages of vital information about health, with over 420 footnotes that include clinical studies and other medical information that support his statements.

UnCreating Dis-ease – Describes how we create and un-create dis-ease. It reveals clearly why modern cancer treatments fail and what is needed to transmute cancer or any dis-ease into vibrant health and opportunity. Every page is full of stimulating and revealing information. Publication projected for late 2002.

The Liver - The Vital Organ – Almost every dis-ease is related to the liver. It is an atrocity that the liver receives such little attention in medical practice, for it is one of the great keys to overcoming dis-ease and obtaining vibrant health. This booklet reveals Dr. Anderson's secrets for cleansing the liver of fats, toxins, and even emotions.

Dramatic Signs of Healing – 32 pages. Explains the healing crisis and cleansing reactions in detail. Highly stimulating. Also includes detailed suggestions for overcoming many crises that people experience. It is an eye-opening and invaluable booklet.

More Recommended Reading

Cherie Soria, *Angel Foods: Healthy Recipes For Heavenly Bodies* – Outstanding and beautifully illustrated cookbook for both exceptional raw and cooked food.

Christine Dreher, *The Cleanse Cookbook* – Excellent cookbook for those who cleanse and want to keep their bodies clean and alkaline.

Dr. Robert Mendelsohn, *Confessions of a Medical Heretic* – A book everyone should read, written by a well-known and respected medical doctor who "just plain had had enough," and clearly revealed the truth about conventional medicine. It's shocking, enlightening, and fun to read.

Dr. Bernard Jensen, *Doctor-Patient Handbook* – A classic 79-page book that clearly explains the healing crisis and many other important points about health and cleansing.

The Disciple John, *The Essene Gospel Of Peace* – The pure, original words of Jesus are translated directly from the Aramaic tongue spoken by Jesus and his disciple John. This is the first of a series smuggled out of the Vatican in the mid-1930's. Jesus discusses health and healing.

Unknown Author, *The Gospel of Perfection also known as The Gospel of the Holy Twelve* – The life of Jesus of Nazareth in a gospel form, and perhaps the most authentic New Testament available. It clearly reveals that Jesus was a strict vegetarian, and that he taught reincarnation and other truths that are more in alignment with Buddhism than with present-day Christianity. This manuscript was known by early Church fathers and purportedly was used by Saint Francis. It is claimed that this manuscript was rediscovered in the late 16th century in Tibet.

Lynes., Barry, *The Healing of Cancer, The Cures - the Cover-Up and the Solution Now!* – If you would like a concise history of what conventional medicine, the FDA, AMA, and our government does to suppress truth and cures, to control people, and to make more money, read this. Very enlightening.

Dr. Candace Pert, *Molecules of Emotion* – Science at the highest level proves that emotions actually do control our bodies, and especially the immune system. Well written and very interesting.

Jamey Dina and Kim Sproul, *Uncooking with Jamey and Kim* – More than 100 raw-food recipes, including pizza, sweet rolls, pies, etc.

Ehret, Professor Arnold, *Mucusless Diet Healing System* – Achieve excellent health via diet and cleansing, and find out why it works so well. Gives excellent guidelines on eating. Very popular book.

Ehret, Professor Arnold, *Rational Fasting* – One of the very best books about water fasting, with instructions.

Griffin, Edward, *World Without Cancer* – A shocking book about what is really behind conventional medicine. Find out about the Allied bombing of Berlin in W.W. II, when the only buildings left standing were those owned by the drug cartels. Guess who built trucks for the Nazis and the Americans during the war. What does this have to do with medical drugs? Learn just how far medical authorities will go to cover up a cure for cancer.

Other Recommended Books

The Secret Teachings of Jesus – Four Gnostic Gospels, Includes: The Gospel of Thomas, The Secret Book of James, The Book of Thomas, and The Secret Book of John – This is part of the Nag Hammadi manuscripts found in Egypt in 1945. Available through Mt. Shasta Herb & Health, 108 Chestnut St., Mt. Shasta, CA, 96067, (530) 926-0633 – toll free (888) 343-7225, http://www.shastaspirit.com/herbhealth/

Cleansing, Fasting, and Diet

Dr. Bernard Jensen, *Tissue Cleansing Through Bowel Management.* Escondido, California: Bernard Jensen Publishing, 1981.

Phillip Partee, *Fasting and Losing Weight.* Sarasota, Florida: United Press Publication, Inc., 1979.

Garbriel Cousens, M.D., *Conscious Eating.* Patagonia, Arizona: Essene Vision Books, 1992.

Barbara Parham. *What's Wrong with Eating Meat?* Denver, Colorado: Ananda Marga Publications, 1979.

John Robbins. *Diet for a New America.* Walpole, New Hampshire: Stillpoint Publishing, 1987.

Marcia Madhuri Acciardo, *Light Eating for Survival.* 21st Century Publications, P.O. Box 702, Fairfield, Louisiana 52556

Ann Wigmore, *Recipes for Longer Life.* Wayne, New Jersey: Avery Publishing Group, 1978.

Harvey and Marilyn Diamond, *Fit for Life.* NewYork, New York: Warner Books, 1985.

Viktoras Kulvinskas, M.S., *Love Your Body* Publication – *Live Food Recipes.* Woodstock Valley, Connecticut: Omangod Press, 1972.

Bernard Jensen, Ph.D., *Juicing Therapy.* Escondido, California: Bernard Jensen Publishing, 1992.

pH

Ted M. Morter, Jr., B.S., M.A., D.C., *An Apple a Day?*, Rogers, Arkansas: B.E.S.T. Research, Inc., 1996. (800) 874-1478.

Ted M. Morter, Jr. B.S., M.A., D.C., *Correlative Urinalysis.* Rogers, Arkansas: B.E.S.T. Research Inc., 1987.

Herman Aihara, *Acid and Alkaline*. Oroville, California: George Ohsawa Macrobiotic Foundation, 1986.

Vaccines

Hannah Allen, *Don't Get Stuck: The Case Against Vaccinations*. Tampa, Florida: American Natural Hygiene Society, 1985.

Harris L. Coulter, and Barbara Loe Fisher, *A Shot in the Dark: Why the P in DPT Vaccination May Be Hazardous to Your Child's Health*. Garden City Park, New York: Avery Publishing Group, Inc., 1991.

Robert Mendelsohn, M.D., *But Doctor, About That Shot – The Risks of Immunizations and How to Avoid Them*. Evanston, Illinois: "The People's Doctor Newsletter," 1988.

The Randolph Society, Inc., *The Dangers of Immunization*. Quakerstown, Pennsylvania: The Randolph Society, Inc, 1987.

Eleanor McBean, Ph.D., *The Poisoned Needle – Is Polio Vaccine Necessary?* Mokelumne Hill, California: Health Research, 1959.

Eleanor McBean, Ph.D., *Vaccinations Do Not Protect*. Manachaca, Texas: Health Excellence Systems, 1991.

Elben, *Vaccination Condemned - Book One*. Los Angeles, California: Better Life Research, 1981.

Harris L. Coulter, *Vaccination, Social Violence, and Criminality: The Medical Assault on the American Brain*. Berkeley, California: North Altantic Books, 1990.

Neil Z. Miller. *Vaccines: Are They Really Safe and Effective? A Parent's Guide To Childhood Shots*. Santa Fe, New Mexico: New Atlantan Press, 1992.

M. Beddow Bayly. *The Case Against Vaccination*. London: William H. Taylor and Sons, Ltd. Printers, 1936.

James Walene. *Immunization: The Reality Behind the Myth*. South Hadley, Massachusetts: Bergin & Garvey, 1988.

Richard Moskowitz, M.D., *The Case Against Immunizations*. Washington, D.C.: National Center for Homeopathy, 1983.

Tom Finn, Esq. *Dangers of Compulsory Immunizations – How to Avoid Them Legally*. New Port Richey, Florida: Family Fitness Press, 1988.

Hoffman & Chriss Buttram M.D., *Vaccinations & Immune Malfunctions*, Quakerstown: Humanitarian Publications Co., Pennsylvania, 1982.

Isaac Golden, Ph.D. *Vaccination? A Review of Risks and Alternatives*, 4th edition. Geelong, Victoria, Canada: Aurum Healing Centre, 1993.

Medical Conspiracy

Elaine Feuer, *Innocent Casualties – The FDA's War Against Humanity*. Pittsburgh, Pennsylvania: Dorrance Publishing Co., Inc., 1996.

Eustace Mullins, *Murder By Injection, The Story of the Medical Conspiracy Against America*. Staunton, Virginia: The National Council for Medical Research, 1988.

Ralph W. Moss, *The Cancer Industry – Unravelling the Politics*. New York, New York: Paragon House, 1989.

Harvey Diamond, *A Case Against Medicine*. Santa Monica, Calfironia: Golden Glow Publishers, 1979

Morris A. Bealle, *The Drug Story*. Spanish Fork, Utah: The Hornet's Nest, 1976.

Robert Mendelsohn, M.D., MALE *PRACTICE - How Doctors Manipulate Women*. Don Mills, Ontario, Canada: Beaverbooks, Ltd., 1981.

Paul Sitt, *Fighting the Food Giants*. Denver, Colorado: Nutri-Books, 1980.

Dr. John Yiamouyiannis, *Fluoride The Aging Factor*. Delaware, Ohio: Health Action Press, 1993.

Alan Cantwell Jr., M.D., *AIDS and the Doctors of Death*. Los Angeles, California: Aries Rising Press, 1988.

Guylaine Lanctot, M.D., *The Medical Mafia*. Coaticook, Quebec, Canada: Here's The Key Inc., 1995.

Charles B. Inlander, President, People's Medical Society, Lowell S. Levin, Professor, Yale University School of Medicine, Ed Weiner Senior Editor, People's Medical Society, *Medicine On Trial - The Appalling Story of Ineptitude, Malfeasance, Neglect, and Arrogance*. New York, New York: Prentice Hall Press, 1988.

P. J. Lisa, *Are You a Target for Elimination?* Huntington Beach, California: International Institute of Natural Health Sciences, Inc.,1984.

Silver- Mercury Amalgam Fillings

H.L. Queen, *Chronic Mercury Toxicity*. Colorado Springs, Colorado: Queen and Company, Health Communication, Inc., 1988.

Hal A. Huggins, DDS, *It's All in Your Head – Dis-eases Caused By Silver-Mercury Fillings*. New York, New York: Avery Press, 1993.

Weston Price, D.D.S., M.S., *The Price of Root Canals*. The author directed the Research Institute of the National Dental Association for 14 years. Find out how root canals kill, and cause serious dis-ease. This book is available from Dr. Huggins' office at (719) 522-0566 in Colorado Springs, Colorado.

BIBLIOGRAPHY

Alexandersson, Olof. *Living Water: Viktor Schauberger and the Secrets of Natural Energy.* Bath, UK: Gateway Books, 1982. Distributed by The Great Tradition, Lower Lake, California.

Allen, Ph.D., Lindsay H.; Oddoye, Ph.D., E.A.; and Margen, M.D., S. "Salt-Sensitive Essential Hypercalciuria; A Longer Term Study." *The American Journal of Clinical Nutrition,* 1979; April; Issue 32, pg. 741-749.

American Iatrogenic Association's Home Page – (http://www.aia.iatrogenic.org) American Iatrogenic Association, 2513 S. Gessner, #232, Houston, Texas 77063.

Anderson, N.D., N.M.D. Rich, *Cleanse and Purify Thyself,* Book 2. Mt. Shasta, California: Christobe Publishing, 2000.

---. *UnCreating Dis-ease.* Mt. Shasta, California: Christobe Publishing, projected publication 2001.

"Autism and Microorganisms." Videotape Series: Tape 1. William Shaw, Ph.D. Produced by the Great Plains Laboratory, Overland Park, Kansas. Phone 913-341-8949.

Boik, John. *Cancer & Natural Medicine.* Princeton, Minnesota: Oregon Medical Press, 1996. E-mail [ompress@sherbtel.net] Web Site (http://www.teleport.com/~ormed)

Brennan, T. A; Leap, L. L.; Liard, N. M.; Herbert, L.; Localio, A. R.; Lawthers, A. G.; Newhouse, J. P.; Weiler, P. C.; Hiatt, H. H. "Incidence of Adverse Event and Negligence in Hospitalized Patients. Results of the Harvard Medical Practice Study." *New England Journal of Medicine,* 1991; Feb. 7, pg. 370-376.

Burr, M. L.; and Sweetnam, P. M. "Vegetarianism, Dietary Fiber, and Mortality." *American Journal of Clinical Nutrition,* 1982; Nov.; Vol. 36, pg. 873-877.

Clark, B.S., M.D., Ph.Sa., P. L. *How to Live and Eat for Health,* 5th Edition. Chicago, Illinois: The Health School, 1929.

Coulter, Harris L. *Vaccination, Social Violence, and Criminality: The Medical Assault on the American Brain*. Berkeley, California: North Atlantic Books, 1990.

Fife, N.D., Bruce. *The Healing Crisis*. Colorado Springs, Colorado: HealthWise Publications, 1997.

The Gospel of the Perfect Life, Mt. Shasta, California: Christobe Publishing, projected publication 2001.

Gray, Dr. Robert. *The Colon Health Handbook*. Reno, Nevada: Emerald Publishing, 1986.

Guyton, A.C. *Textbook of Medical Physiology*, 7th edition. Philadelphia, Pennsylvania: W. B. Saunders Co, 1986.

"Health Costs Soaring." *USA Today*," 1991; Dec. 30; Monday.

Irons, Sr., Victor Earl. *The Destruction of Your Own Natural Protective Mechanism*. Kansas City, Missouri: V.E. Irons, Inc., 1995. (800) 544-8147.

Jensen, D.C., N.D., Ph.D, Bernard. *Doctor-Patient Handbook*. Escondido, California: Bernard Jensen Publishing, 1976.

---. *Iridology, The Science and Practice in the Healing Arts*, Volume II. Escondido, California: Bernard Jensen Publications, 1982.

---. *Tissue Cleansing Through Bowel Management*. Escondido, California: Bernard Jensen Publications, 1981.

Journal of Community Health, 1980; Spring; Vol.5, No. 3., pg. 149-158. Note: Figures after 1980 have not been released.

Kapit, Wynn; Macey, Robert; and Meisami, Esmail. *The Physiology Coloring Book*. Philadelphia, Pennsylvania: Harper Collins Publishers, 1987.

Kervran, Professor C. Lewis. *Biological Transmutations*. Magalia, California: Happiness Press, 1988.

Kurtz; M.D., Theodore W.; Al-Bander, M.D., Hamoundi A.; Morris, Jr., M.D., R. Curtis. "Salt-Sensitive Essential Hypertension In Men." *New England Journal of Medicine,* Vol. 317, No. 17, pg. 1043-1048.

Lanctot, M.D., Guylaine. *The Medical Mafia*. Coaticook, Quebec, Canada: Here's The Key, Inc., 1995.

Lee, M.D., Richard; Bithell, M.D., Thomas; Forester, M.D., John; Athens, M.D., John; Lukens, M.D., John. *Wintrobe's Clinical Hematology.* Philadelphia, Pennsylvania: Lea & Febiger, 1993.

Malstrom, N.D., M.T., Stan. "Your Colon: Its Character, Care and Therapy." Orem, Utah: BiWorld Publications, Inc., 1981.

Mendelsohn, M.D., Robert S. *Confessions of a Medical Heretic.* Chicago, Illinois: Contemporary Books, 1979.

Mindell, Ph.D., Earl , The Web Page (http://www.drearlmindell.com).

National Center for Health Statistics through the U.S. Department of Health & Human Services Center for Dis-ease Control, Statistical Reports.

Pert, Ph.D., Candace B. *Molecules of Emotion: The Science Behind Mind-Body Medicine.* New York, New York: Touchstone, 1999.

Poley, J. Ranier. "The Scanning Electron Microscope: How Valuable in the Evaluation of Small Bowel Mucosal Pathology in Chronic Childhood Diarrhea?" *Journal of Pediatric Gastroenterology and Nutrition,* 1991; May-June; 7(3), pg. 386-394.

N. Rangavajhyala, K. M. Shahani, G. Sridevi, and S. Srikumaran. "Nonlipopolysaccharide Component(s) of *Lactobacillus acidophilus* Stimulate(s) the Production of Interleukin-a and Tumor Necrosis Factor-q by Murine Macrophages." *Nutrition and Cancer,* Vol. 27 or 28 (2), pg. 130-134.

Rose, W. C. *Physiology Review,* 1938; Vol. 18, pg. 109-136.

Schmidt, Gerald K.; and Roberts, Larry S. *Foundations of Parasitology.* St. Louis, Missouri: Times Mirror/Mosby College Publishing, 1989.

Shahani, Khem M.; Vakie, Jayanthkumar R.; and Chandan, Rarnesh Chandra. United States Patent #3,689,640. September 5, 1972.

Shahani, K. M.; Vakie, J. R.; and Kilara, A. "Natural Antibiotic Activity of *Lactobacillus acidophilus* and *bulgaricus.*" Department of Food Sciences and Technology, University of Nebraska, Lincoln, Nebraska 68583.

Shils, Maurice E.; and Young, Vernon R. *Modern Nutrition in Health and Dis-ease,* 7th Edition. Philadelphia, Pennsylvania: Lea & Febiger, 1988.

Smith, B. L. "Organic Foods vs. Supermarket Foods; Element Levels." *Journal of Applied Nutrition*, 1993; Vol. 45, No. 1, pg. 35-39.

Szekely, Edmond Bordeaux, ed.; as recorded by John, the Disciple of Jesus Christ. *The Essene Gospel of Peace.* Nelson, British Columbia, Canada: International Biogenic Society, 1981.

The Secret Teachings Of Jesus: Four Gnostic Gospels. Translated by Marvin W. Meyer. New York, New York: Random House, 1984.

The Gospel of the Perfect Life. Mt. Shasta, California: Christobe Publishing, projected publication, 2001.

Weiss, Rick, "Correctly Prescribed Drugs Take Heavy Toll." *The Washington Post*, 1998; April 15, pg. A-1.

Yamada, T., ed. *Textbook of Gastroenterology.* Philadelphia, Pennsylvania: J. P. Lippincott Co., 1991.

INDEX